PRINCIPLES OF TIBETAN MEDICINE

Principles of
TIBETAN MEDICINE

Tibetan Medicine is a traditional systems of medicine which has been practised for over 2500 years, Tibetan medicine originates from the pre-Buddhist Bon era of Tibetan History, During this time there was extensive medical knowledge in Tibet and medical study was based on the four Bon medical texts known as gSo-rig Bhoom-Shi.

Principles of
TIBETAN MEDICINE

Dr. Tamdin Sither Bradley

MOTILAL BANARSIDASS
INTERNATIONAL
DELHI

Reprint Edition : Delhi, 2023, 2024
First Indian Edition : Delhi, 2010

ISBN : 978-81-19394-10-4

Also available at
MOTILAL BANARSIDASS INTERNATIONAL
H. O.- 41 U.A. Bungalow Road, (Back Lane)Jawahar Nagar, Delhi - 110 007
4261 (basement) Lane #3, Ansari Road, Darya Ganj, New Delhi - 110 002
203 Royapettah High Road, Mylapore, Chennai - 600 004
12/1A, 2nd Floor, Bankim Chatterjee Street, Kolkata - 700 073
Stockist : Motilal Books, Ashok Rajpath, Near Kali Mandir, Patna - 800 004

For Sale in Asia Only

Printed in India
MOTILAL BANARSIDASS INTERNATIONAL

CONTENTS

	Acknowledgements	vi
	Dedication	vii
1	History of Tibetan Medicine	1
2	*gso-ba Rig-pa* – The Science of Healing	5
3	The Theory of Tibetan Medicine	11
4	Causative Factors of Illness	22
5	Human Anatomy and Physiology	42
6	Common Diseases and Illnesses	59
7	Methods of Diagnosis	81
8	Treatment Techniques – Part I	108
9	Treatment Techniques – Part II	142
10	Case Histories	179
11	The Practising Physician	184
	Final Thoughts	190
	Resources	191

ACKNOWLEDGEMENTS

My sincere thanks to the Tibetan Medical and Astrological Institute for giving me the opportunity to study Tibetan medicine. To all my teachers of past and present for guiding me to the right path – the late Professor Bashi Phuntsok Wangyal, Dr Tenzin Choedrak, Dr Pasang Yonten Arya, Dr Lobsang Chophel, Dr Kunga Gyurmey Nyarongsher, Gen. Gendhun Jinpa, Gen. Dorjee Gyalpo and the late Gen. Nyima Tsering.

To all my friends and colleagues through the years who have helped to promote Tibetan medicine. To Mr Tseten Samdup from Office of Tibet, London.

To all the editorial staff at Thorsons for their help and assistance.

To my family for their support and encouragement. To my husband Philip for his assistance and his perseverance which enabled me to finish everything on time.

Lastly to my greatest inspiration, my uncle, the monk Gen. Tsultrim Sangpo, without whose guidance I would never have been a physician.

DEDICATION

This book is dedicated to all my patients.

1

HISTORY OF TIBETAN MEDICINE

Methods for keeping healthy and promoting longevity have been present in Tibet for many thousands of years. For example, Tibetans know that drinking hot water will relieve indigestion and placing melted butter in cuts and wounds will stop bleeding and promote healing.

Tibetan medicine is a traditional system of medicine which has been practised for over 2500 years. Tibetan medicine originates from the pre-Buddhist Bon era of Tibetan history. During this time there was extensive medical knowledge in Tibet and medical study was based on the four Bon medical texts known as *gSo-rig Bhoom-Shi*. This period in Tibetan medical history lasted from sixth century BC to seventh century AD.

However, in the seventh century changes were brought about and the influence of other medical systems became incorporated into Tibetan medical knowledge. During the reign of King Songsten Gampo the first international conference on Tibetan medicine was held in Samye in Tibet. Songsten Gampo invited to this conference many physicians from neighbouring countries such as Persia, India and China. In the eighth century, during the reign of King Trisong Detsen, Buddhism replaced

Bon as the state religion of Tibet. This led to the suppression of Bon religion, culture and medical knowledge in Tibet.

In 762 Yuthog Yongten Gonpo, the court physician to Trisong Detsen, established the first Tibetan medical college in Tibet in Kongpo, the valley of medicine. Here he systematized the *gSo-rig Bhoom-Shi* into the nine wordings in a single sentence and replaced the old Bon titles and conclusions with Buddhist ones. During this time he added medical knowledge from neighbouring countries such as India and China. His work is the basis for the *rGyud-bzhi* – the four Tibetan medical tantras.

There are many books which state that Tibetan medical knowledge is solely derived from India and China. This is not true as Tibet has had its own medical knowledge for thousands of years and it is important to remember that the Bon and Buddhist eras comprise two different historical periods of Tibet.

In the twelfth century Yuthog the Younger further researched and edited the *rGyud-bzhi*. This version has remained to this day the standard and most authoritative of Tibetan medical texts. It continues to be studied and practised by Tibetan physicians.

In the fifteenth century the Tibetan medical system divided itself into two main schools, the *Jangpa* and the *Zurpa*. In the seventeenth century the Fifth Dalai Lama was a great patron of Tibetan medicine, and his regent, Sangye Gyamtso, was a great Tibetan physician and scholar who wrote the commentary on the four medical tantras which is known as the Blue Beryl. In 1696 the Chagpori College of Medicine was founded by the Fifth Dalai Lama. In 1916 the Thirteenth Dalai Lama founded the Men-Tsee-Kang School of Medicine and Astrology in Lhasa, Tibet.

After the Tibetan uprising in 1959 Tibetans went into exile in India and in 1961, under the initiative of His Holiness the Fourteenth Dalai Lama, the Tibetan Government in Exile established the Tibetan Medical Centre in Dharamsala, India. This

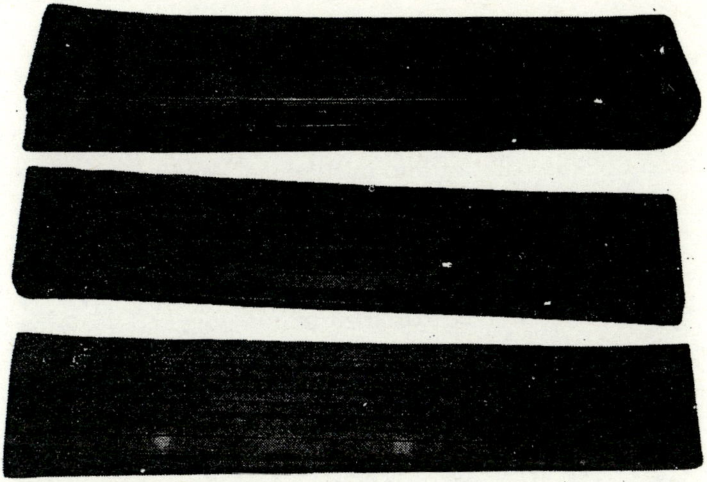

The rGyud-bzhi – The four medical tantras

was built up by the hard work of doctors such as Dr Yeshi Dhonden and the late Dr Jamyang Tashi Tsona, both of whom were physicians to His Holiness. Since 1982 Tibetan medicine has expanded greatly due to Dr Tenzin Choedak (the senior physician to His Holiness the Dalai Lama) coming to India from Tibet and bringing with him a vast and profound Tibetan medical knowledge, especially with regard to Tibetan pharmaceutical formulae.

At present there are over 50 branch clinics of the Tibetan Medical and Astrological Institute as well as many private clinics in India, Nepal and a few doctors in Europe, such as myself, who also have private practices. From 1962 to 1995 there have been 153 Tibetan doctors who have successfully qualified from the Tibetan Medical and Astrological Institute and of these 54 were women. Since 1979 even in Tibet the communist Chinese have revived Tibetan medicine despite the fact they have no respect whatsoever for Tibet's religion and culture. Neverthless, they have opened many clinics and places for study such as the Lhasa Men-Tsee-Kang. For the Chinese seeing is believing.

In 1998 the first International Congress on Tibetan Medicine was held outside Tibet in Washington DC where over 200 Tibetan doctors, Tibetan Buddhist lamas, Western doctors, scientists and psychologists participated. Opened by His Holiness the Dalai Lama the Congress was a great success and there will now be a second Congress in 2001. As a guest speaker at this congress I found it to be extremely stimulating and inspiring to be able to share our unique medical knowledge with the rest of the world.

2

GSO-BA RIG-PA – THE SCIENCE OF HEALING

Tibetan medicine is a complete medical system. It is one of the oldest surviving forms of ancient medicine and it has been in use for over 2500 years. For many centuries Tibetan medicine has been successfully practised in Tibet, China, Mongolia, Buddhist regions of Russia and Central Asia, and the Himalayan kingdoms of Nepal, Sikkim, Bhutan, Ladakh and Northern India.

It is called *gSo-ba Rig-pa,* or the science of healing, and is based on the four medical tantras called *rGyud-bzhi*. These are the root tantra, explanatory tantra, instructional tantra and the subsequent tantra. The root tantra which contains six chapters, gives an overall view of the *rGyud-bzhi;* the explanatory tantra contains thirty-one chapters and explains and describes in detail the human body, including embryology, anatomy and physiology; the instructional tantra contains ninety-two chapters dealing with the causes, symptoms and treatment of many different kinds of diseases; the subsequent tantra contains twenty-five chapters which deal with diagnosis and pharmacology. In addition to the four tantras there are two concluding chapters which condense all the preceding information. This gives a total of 156 chapters with 5900 verses.

To be a fully qualified Tibetan physician we have to study these four medical tantras for a minimum of seven years. The first four years are spent studying the Tibetan medical texts where we have to memorize approximately forty specific chapters. One month each year is also spent collecting herbs in the Himalayas. In addition to studying the medical texts we also have to study Tibetan linguistics, grammar, poetry and have a complete understanding of basic Tibetan Buddhist teachings contained in works such as Shantideva's *Guide to the Bodhisattva's Way of Life*. In the fifth year we have to take both oral and written exams on the four medical tantras and at the end of the fifth year we take the Medicine Buddha initiation both as a blessing and in order to enhance our powers of healing as practitioners of Tibetan medicine. Like a beautiful woman for whom jewels and fine clothes merely magnifies and reinforces her beauty, so the initiation magnifies and reinforces the healing powers of the practitioner. The sixth and seventh years are spent at a branch clinic of the Tibetan Medical and Astrological Institute where practical training is given in pulse reading, urinalysis and dealing with patients.

Compared to other forms of alternative medicine in the West, Tibetan medicine is very new and this is because there are very few fully qualified Tibetan doctors here; there are no more than eight of us in both Europe and the United States. The uniqueness of Tibetan medicine is that it is based on Buddhist philosophical principles, astrology and the close relationship between the mind and body. The basic principle of Tibetan medicine is balancing the three principal energies or *Nyes-pa-gsum*. The three principal energies are *Loong, mKhris-pa* and *Bad-Kan*.

Loong (pronounced as *loong*) is the subtle flow of energy which circulates throughout our body and aids all movements and activities connected with mind, speech and body. ***mKhris-pa*** (pronounced as *tree –pa*) is heat energy which circulates throughout our body and balances bodily temperature, digestion and vitality. ***Bad-Kan*** (pronounced as *Beh – ken*) is a fluid energy which circulates throughout our body. It keeps our joints flexible and aids the functioning of bodily stability and the lymphatic system.

These Tibetan terms are being left as they are throughout this book as there are no equivalent translations in English for them. Therefore if you wish to understand the explanation of Tibetan medicine given in this book, it is very important to get used to the terms *Loong*, *mKhris-pa* and *Bad-Kan*.

When the three principal energies are in balance we are healthy and when they are out of balance we are sick. In the Tibetan medical texts the main long-term cause of illnesses and suffering is *ma-rig-pa*, or ignorance. This ignorance generates in turn the three poisons of desire, anger and closed-mindedness. The short-term causes are improper diet, unwholesome lifestyle and seasonal factors. A combination of these causes makes us sick and the physician first has to diagnose the illness through questioning and listening with a sympathetic ear. The physician then makes an overall observation of the patient, especially through tongue diagnosis and urinalysis (in which the practitioner looks at the colour, smell, bubbles, steam and sediments of the urine). Finally the physician reads the pulse of the patient, and for the Tibetan physician pulse reading is a great source of information.

Once diagnosis is made treatment can begin. The main aim of the treatment is to balance and correct the three principal energies. For example, if one of the energies is in excess treatment is given to decrease it or if one of the energies is deficient treatment is given to increase it. Tibetan medicine is not based on any magic, mystery or miracle cures, rather it is based on an ancient system of medicine which has been passed down from generation to generation. Tibetan medicine today is the culmination of the experience and knowledge of enlightened physicians through the course of many centuries – just like honey collected in a pot cannot be produced from a single flower but is the sum of many flowers. There is no end to knowledge, and with the continual arising of new diseases Tibetan medical research goes on, and at the Tibetan Medical and Astrological Institute there is a research department producing new forms of Tibetan medicine aimed at treating modern diseases.

The Tibetan physician aims to treat the patient first of all through dietary advice according to each individual's body constitution, and through advice on leading a wholesome lifestyle. If this is not enough, medicine is prescribed. Tibetan pharmacology is extremely rich in both depth and variety. It makes use of gems, minerals, metals, soils, saps, woods and herbal plants. Medicines can be a combination of as little as three ingredients or as many as 157. At present there are approximately 250 different types of medicine which are manufactured. One of these preparations is a medicine called *Padma 28* and this is now commercially available. Middlesex hospital in London has performed clinical trials on it and it has proven to be effective for vascular diseases (a condition caused by hardening of the arteries in the legs) and there is the possibility it will help in the treatment of hepatitis B and C. When one considers that there are 250 other forms of Tibetan medicine to be explored it gives great hope for the potential of Tibetan medicine to help as many people as possible. Performing or physical therapies are used as a last resort in Tibetan medicine. At present we use moxibustion, cupping and golden needle therapy.

There is also an advanced form of Tibetan meditation known as *tomo* yoga which is practised by training the subtle flow of *Loong* energy. At the International Congress on Tibetan Medicine the researcher Herbert Benson from Harvard Medical

School gave a slide show of Tibetan monks practising *tomo* yoga. Dr Charles Raison from the University of California commented that *tomo* meditation may offer more understanding about depression and open up the possibility of non-pharmacological self-help. The monks were meditating in conditions just a few degrees above freezing yet they were able to completely dry wet sheets that were wrapped around them. Researchers from the University of California in San Francisco have also discovered that raising the peripheral skin temperature during deep meditation accelerates the healing of wounds just as effectively as the use of antibiotics.

Astrology is also connected to Tibetan medicine. It is considered in the preparation of certain special medicines, during the time of herb collection and when performing therapies such as moxibustion. All medicines are then blessed and consecrated according to Tibetan Buddhist rituals. When I was studying at the Tibetan Medical College and also working at the Tibetan Medical and Astrological Institute clinic, we would recite the Medicine Buddha prayers and mantra every morning before we began our day.

Tibetan medicine is beneficial for chronic diseases such as digestive problems, arthritis, asthma, skin problems, problems related to the liver and kidneys, sinus problems, insomnia, anxiety, heart disease and problems related to the central nervous system. Tibetan *gSo-ba Rig-pa* also treats the roots of the disease and not just the symptoms. The Tibetan medical texts give the following example: A failure to treat the roots or the cause of the disease is the same as having a poisonous tree and just cutting off the leaves and branches without pulling it out from its roots; if you just cut the leaves and branches the tree will still continue to grow.

A real-life example is a patient of mine who suffered bad migraines. She had been taking painkillers which helped, but when the effects wore off she needed to take more of them. My diagnosis upon seeing her was that she was suffering from chronic constipation and therefore I prescribed medicine to clear it. This was the root of her problem. As a result of treating her constipation, her migraines were reduced over time. If a person is suffering from a chronic disease and expects a quick solution through taking Tibetan medicine, this will not be possible. The patient has to be prepared to take the medicine over a period of time before its positive results will show.

In the West there are many people at present who wish to study Tibetan medicine, but unfortunately the four medical tantras have not been translated into English. This problem is no doubt exacerbated by the fact that Tibetans no longer have their own country where the proper facilities for such works would have existed. The contents of the four medical tantras are extremely condensed and just one sentence could take pages to be fully explained. To be successfully and accurately translated would require a group of people who have studied the four medical tantras and who also have perfect knowledge of English. It is vital there is no misunderstanding of the medical terms and that the meaning of the four medical tantras are not diluted in any way.

Tibetan medical knowledge is not just for the benefit of Tibetans but for the rest of the world. There is no doubt that practitioners of Tibetan medicine can learn a great deal from allopathic forms of medicine, and similarly Western medical practitioners can learn and benefit from *gSo-ba Rig-pa*. Both medicines are based on the same concepts of healing and relief of suffering.

3

THE THEORY OF TIBETAN MEDICINE

The theory of Tibetan medicine is to keep in balance the three principal energies or *Nyes-pa-gsum*. In the *rGyud-bzhi* (the four medical tantras) it says that the three principal energies are like three brothers; if one brother has a problem it is impossible for the other brothers to relax or feel comfortable. Therefore it is very important for the three principal energies to be in a state of equilibrium in order for our mind and body to function properly.

Let us first look in more detail at the three principal energies. They are *Loong*, *mKhris-pa* and *Bad-Kan*.

LOONG

What is *Loong*? In Tibetan *Loong* means mobility. This subtle flow of energy circulates throughout our body carrying blood and nutrients. It also helps the respiratory system, sensory organs and bodily growth. It separates nutrients and waste products in our body. The main function of *Loong*, however, is to carry the movements of mind, speech and body. Movements and activities such as stretching and walking are performed by this energy. Just because this subtle energy cannot be seen under the microscope does not mean that it is not there; we cannot see the wind or air, but are still able to feel it when it touches our skin and able to see it when branches and leaves sway in the breeze. *Loong* is very much connected to the air element.

When *Loong* is in excess, deficient or blocked in our body, we will suffer from sleeplessness, aches and pains in the bones, dry skin, colon upsets, anxiety and palpitations. *Loong* is connected with the heart, large intestines, lungs, blood vessels and the nerves. We can detect the imbalance of this subtle flow of energy through various methods of diagnosis, especially when treating patients suffering from insomnia, heart disease and problems related to the central nervous system.

From my own experience the majority of people who come to see me in England (where I practise) suffer from *Loong*-related problems. In this regard I believe Tibetan medicine can be very beneficial and can treat many modern diseases such as MS, blood pressure disorders or Parkinson's disease. All of these conditions have their origin in an imbalance of *Loong* and cannot be treated adaquately by allopathic medicine.

In the *rGyud-bzhi* there are 63 different types of *Loong*-related diseases; in this book I am just going to describe the five main types.

FIVE TYPES OF LOONG

Loong Srog-dzin is known as the life-grasping *Loong*. This *Loong* is located in the brain and it moves from the pharynx down to the oesophagus. Its function is to help the swallowing of food, spitting, sneezing, eructation, inhalation and to focus the mind. An imbalance of *Loong Srog-dzin* can be caused when the mind is focused too much when meditating without proper instruction, or when thinking obsessively about one particular subject or object. At its most pronounced it can lead to insanity. This is why in the Tibetan community, where there are many practitioners of meditation, everyone knows what *Loong Srog-dzin* is. Consequently if a practitioner suffers from *Loong Srog-dzin* people believe that they have not been meditating according to the proper instructions.

Loong Gyen-rgyu is known as the upward moving *Loong*. This *Loong* is located in the thorax and it moves in the nose, tongue and throat. Its function is to help speech, clarity of memory and mental diligence. When *Loong Gyen-rgyu* is disturbed it affects our speech.

Loong Khyab-byed is known as all-pervading *Loong*. This *Loong* is located in the heart and is responsible for blood circulation and the carrying of nutrients throughout the body. It helps us in walking, lifting, stretching, the contraction of limbs and the opening and closing of our mouth and eyes. When there is an imbalance in *Loong Khyab-byed* it affects all bodily movements and motor functions and is the cause of heart disease. As it is all-pervading, *Loong Khyab-byed* plays a very important role in the proper functioning of our mind and body.

Loong Me-mnyam is known as fire-accompanying *Loong*. This *Loong* is located in the stomach and it moves in the small intestine and the large intestine. It helps to separate nutrients and waste products, promotes digestion and helps the process of the seven bodily constituents. When there is an imbalance in *Loong Me-mnyam* it can affect the whole of the digestive system.

Loong Thur-sel is known as downward cleansing *Loong*. This *Loong* is located in the rectum and it flows through the large intestine, bladder, genitalia and the thighs. Its function is to expel faeces, urine, menstruation, semen and the foetus. When there is imbalance in *Loong Thur-sel* it can affect all the eliminating functions of the body, for example during childbirth it can delay the delivery of the baby from the mother's womb.

mKhris-pa

What is *mKhris-pa*? In Tibetan *mKhris-pa* means flame. The main function of *mKhris-pa* is to keep in balance the bodily temperature, to aid digestion and absorption, and to give vitality to the body. *mKhris-pa* is also responsible for us feeling hungry and thirsty at the right times. It gives lustre to the skin, protects us from cold and chills, and mentally it provides us with courage and determination.

If we have too much heat in our body it burns our system, and damages internal organs such as the liver, small intestine and gall bladder. It creates high blood pressure and other blood related problems, it damages eyesight and it causes diarrhoea. If we have too little heat in our body we are always cold and as a result we can feel low self-esteem. Inflammatory illnesses, infections and blood disorders are all connected to an imbalance of *mKhris-pa*. The nature of *mKhris-pa* is hot and it is closely connected with the fire element.

mKhris-pa disorders are very common in countries such as India where the climate is hot. In the *rGyud-bzhi* there are 47 *mKhris-pa* disorders, and here I will describe the five main *mKhris-pas*.

Five Types of mKhris-pa

mKhris-pa Jyoo-byed is known as digesting *mKhris-pa*. It is located in the small intestine and its main function is to digest food and drink. It promotes bodily heat and aids in the functioning of the four other main types of *mKhris-pa*. Disturbance of this *mKhris-pa* can lead to digestive problems such as blood cholesterol and diarrhoea. Proper absorption depends very much on this *mKhris-pa*.

mKhris-pa sGrub-byed, known as accomplishing *mKhris-pa*, is located in the heart and its main function is to motivate our minds. It helps us to succeed in our life-goals and ambitions and in this respect it helps to build up our confidence. Disturbance of the *mKhris-pa sGrub-byed* might indicate that we have lost interest in our life.

MKhris-pa mDangs-sgyur is known as colour changing *mKhris-pa*. It is located in the liver and its main function is to promote and maintain the red colouring of essential nutrients in the blood and muscle tissues. If this *mKhris-pa* is disturbed it means we have a deficiency of blood and as a result we will have skin problems such as lucoderma.

MKhris-pa mThong-byed is known as sight *mKhris-pa*. It is located in the eyes and is responsible for vision. When this *mKhris-pa* is disturbed our eyesight suffers.

MKhris-pa mDog-gsel is known as complexion-clearing *mKhris-pa*. It is located in the skin and its function is to clear and promote skin lustre by giving it a healthy and wholesome colour, therefore if this *mKhris-pa* is disturbed it affects our complexion.

BAD-KAN

What is *Bad-Kan*? In Tibetan *Bad* means earth and *Kan* means water. The main function of *Bad-Kan* is to balance our bodily fluids, help mix food in the stomach, keep the mind stable and lubricate our joints. If there is not enough fluid in our system we become dehydrated and if there is too much fluid we retain it. Both these conditions can then block blood circulation and the subtle flow of *Loong* energy. This, in turn, can lead to problems such as oedema, water retention, excess weight, kidney and digestive problems. All of these are mainly connected to a lack of absorption and an inability to digest foodstuffs and liquids and to turn them into essential nutrients. From my experience I have found these problems to be very common in Western countries, for example when I travel on the train I see many middle-aged women with swollen legs and ankles. This is very much connected with lack of absorption and weak functioning of the kidneys. So the nature of *Bad-Kan* is cold and it is most closely related to the water element. In the *rGyud-bzhi* 43 different types of *Bad-Kan* are mentioned and here I will describe the five main types.

FIVE TYPES OF BAD-KAN

Bad-Kan rTen-byed is known as supporting *Bad-Kan*. Its location is in the thorax and its function is to control our thirst and to help support the other four main types of *Bad-Kan*. When this *Bad-Kan* is disturbed we suffer from excessive thirst.

Bad-Kan Myag-byed is known as mixing *Bad-Kan*. Its location is in the stomach and its function is to break down foodstuffs into a semi-liquid form. This mixing process is a very important part of the digestive system, and if it is not functioning properly undigested food will be seen in stools.

Bad-Kan Myong-byed is known as taste receptor *Bad-Kan*. Its location is on the tongue and its function is to distinguish the six primary tastes of sweet, sour, salty, bitter, pungent and astringent. If this *Bad-Kan* is not functioning properly we lose our sense of taste.

Bad-Kan Tsim-byed is known as satisfying *Bad-Kan*. Its location is in the thalamus and its function is to satisfy the power of the five senses of sight, taste, smell, hearing and touch. If by accident this part of the brain is injured it will affect the functioning of these five senses.

Bad-Kan Byor-byed is known as connecting *Bad-Kan*. Its location is in the joints and its function is in the movement of the joints and movements such as stretching and contracting. When it is not functioning properly it can affect the movement of the body.

This is a brief description of the type, location and function of the *Nyes-pa-gsum* and their main sub-divisions. Once the *Nyes-pa-gsum* are in balance then what we call the seven bodily constituents and three eliminating functions are also in balance.

SEVEN BODILY CONSTITUENTS – LUS-ZUNGS BDHUN

The seven bodily constituents are:

1 Essential nutrients from ingested foodstuffs
2 Blood
3 Muscle tissues
4 Fatty tissues
5 Bone
6 Marrow
7 Regenerative fluid

This is how the process works: When we eat or drink something it goes to the stomach where the *Bad-Kan* will help to mix it, the *mKhris-pa* will help to digest it and the *Loong* will help to separate the essential nutrients from the waste products. The essence of essential nutrients will then form blood, the essence of blood forms muscle tissue, the essence of muscle tissue forms fat, the essence of fat forms bones, the essence of bones forms marrow and the essence of bone marrow forms the regenerative fluid.

THE PROCESS OF THE SEVEN BODILY CONSTITUENTS

The essential nutrients then divide into two:

- The essence of essential nutrients is absorbed through the small intestine to the liver where it produces blood, while the impure parts of the essential nutrients turn into mucus.
- The essence of blood forms muscle tissue while impure blood forms bile in the gall bladder.
- The essence of muscle tissue forms fatty tissue and the impure muscle tissue forms grit in the eyes and wax in the ears.
- The essence of fatty tissue forms bones and the impure fatty tissue forms cellulite and perspiration.
- The essence of bone forms marrow and impure bone forms nail and hair.
- The essence of marrow forms regenerative fluid and the impure marrow turns into bodily oils which lubricate our skin and faeces.

The essence of regenerative fluid forms *dhang*, or vital essence. The *dhang* is located in the heart and circulates with the blood throughout our body. It helps prolong our life, promote the senses and vitality, and in my opinion *dhang* is what comprises our immune system. The impure essence of regenerative fluid is used in the reproductive functions which produce sperm and ovum. In the West there are many men who have a weak sperm count and I think this is due to them eating poor quality food, environmental pollution and also because of their stressful lifestyle; by contrast in the East, problems related to male fertility are few.

THREE ELIMINATING FUNCTIONS

With the waste products there are three eliminating functions of waste:

1 Elimination of faeces
2 Elimination of urine
3 Elimination of perspiration

Faeces helps to retain food in the small and large intestines, otherwise it will leak. Urine helps to bring waste products out of our body. Perspiration cleans the pores and softens the skin.

FUNCTIONING OF THE DIGESTIVE SYSTEM

The above seven bodily constituents and three eliminating functions are dependent on the strength of the rate of metabolism, or in Tibetan, *Me-droy*, which means heat. In Tibetan medicine the most important heat is the digestive heat or the *Phoway-Me-droy*.

First of all the *Loong Srog-dzin* helps the process of swallowing food and drink and pushing it down into the stomach. Here the decomposing *Bad-Kan*, which is located in the stomach, will break down the ingested food into a semi-liquid form. During this process the mixture is turned into froth and its taste is sweet, this is because *Bad-Kan* is generated by the earth and water elements and these generate the sweet taste. If one consumes too much sweet food and drink this stage of the digestive process is delayed, causing, in some instances, diabetes. For this reason Tibetan medicine addresses this part of the digestive process and has been very successful in the treatment of diabetes.

This sweet tasting mixture is then further digested and absorbed by the digestive *mKhris-pa* which is located in the jejumum in the small intestine. The nature of the digestive *mKhris-pa* is hot and this gives the chyme a sour or acidic taste. As with the previous stage, if someone eats too much acidic and spicy foods, it affects this stage of the digestive process and will lead to too much acid in the system, causing ulcers. This is the main stage of digestion and absorption and after this the *Loong*

Me-mnyam will help to separate the nutrients and waste products in our large intestine. During this stage the nutrients and waste products have a bitter taste.

THE PROCESS OF THE THREE ELIMINATING FUNCTIONS

At the end of the digesting process the waste products go to the colon and separate into faeces and urine. The faeces go through the sigmoid colon to the rectum and the urine goes through the kidneys to the urethra and to the urinary bladder.

We can now see how important it is for the digestive system to be strong, and in the Tibetan medical texts it is mentioned that the real physician is someone who can look after the patient's digestive system. For example, if someone goes to a Tibetan physician with an arthritic problem, the physician will prescribe a medicine to be taken in the morning to help restore their digestive system. This is because lack of digestive heat leads to so many other problems, one of which is arthritis. In fact it can be said that every illness is connected to our digestive system. With this in mind I can say with full confidence that Tibetan medicine is of great benefit to someone with chronic digestive related problems.

Recently I read a newspaper article saying that many old people in England die in the winter because of the cold. This is because as we get older our metabolic rate becomes slower in the same way that other parts of our body diminish in strength and become weaker in their functioning. To prevent this and to restore the digestive heat Tibetan medicine has two traditional herbal formulas called *Pomegranate 5* and *Pomegranate Nutrient Restorer*. These can be taken along with eating warm and cooked foods (rather than cold and raw foods) and the metabolic rate will increase as a consequence.

Taking care of our digestion is the key to good health and wellbeing. If what we eat is not digested properly it will either come up through vomiting, go down too quickly causing diarrhoea, or it just stagnate within our digestive system, causing tumours, colon cancer and constipation. In this country constipation is very common, and naturally it is related to digestion. However people are often ashamed to admit they are constipated and thus they suffer great discomfort.

Constipation is caused by eating an excess of processed foods, foods with preservatives and sugar, starchy foods, not eating enough fresh fruit and vegetables and by not following a high fibre diet. It is also caused by mental stress, especially when we are so busy that we do not give ourselves enough time to relax and allow our body's eliminating functions to work properly after eating. When we eat too much sugar, either intentionally or unintentionally (for example baked beans contain sugar) we can also suffer from constant constipation which can leave toxins in our system. These in turn causes parasites in our stomach which can further lead to candida and irritable bowel syndrome. To combat these kinds of illness we need to change our basic eating habits and increase our intake of fresh fruit and vegetables, pulses, and cereals. At the same time we need to reduce our intake of sugar and starchy foods. Once our diet is well-balanced we cease to have constant hunger and craving for food.

This process shows how important it is for *Loong*, *mKhris-pa* and *Bad-Kan* to be kept in balance in order for the seven bodily constituents and the three eliminating functions to function normally and thus keep our mind and body in balance. Proper balance will give us health and longevity to enable us to fully enjoy our lives, allow us to attain material wealth and more importantly it will give us the opportunity to practise a spiritual life. Therefore our health is everything.

4

CAUSATIVE FACTORS OF ILLNESS

There are two main divisions in the causative factors of illness: long-term causative factors and short-term causative factors. This chapter also looks at how disease enters our body and accumulates and how it manifests and causes illnesses.

LONG-TERM CAUSES

The Tibetan medical texts state that the main cause of every type of suffering or illness is *Ma-rig-pa* or ignorance. They say that just as a bird is unable to escape its shadow no matter how high it flies, so are we unable to lose our ignorance which has been with us since our birth. Our basic ignorance generates the three poisons of desire, anger and delusion. This concept clearly shows us how Tibetan medicine is closely connected with Buddhist philosophy.

DESIRE

Desire is like salted water, as we drink more we need more; we are never satisfied with what we have. We have got so many wishes to fulfil and we are always seeking something which we believe will give us permanent happiness. However, lasting happiness is not something which can be gained through material comforts. If this was the case we in the West would have no problems and in comparison to people in the East we would always be happy.

The teachings of Buddhism tell us that everything is impermanent. We Tibetans, for example, have lost our country and when the first exiles escaped across the Himalayas they were unable to bring a single family heirloom. This shows how it is foolish to keep on planning for the distant future when we do not know what will happen the very next day. My mother always used to tell me that one day we have to leave our bodies behind and go into the next world empty-handed and alone.

This sort of basic belief helps Tibetans to appreciate the comforts which we have and to be contented with them. One of my father's friends used to say that as long as we are not in debt we are rich. So basic simplicity in our lives is best. Desire generates greed, and when our wishes are not fulfilled we become restless and suffer from sleeplessness. This causes further anxiety and tension which can disrupt the subtle flow of *Loong* and, in some extreme cases, cause madness. In the Tibetan medical texts desire is symbolized by a bird which is the creature most associated with sex in the animal kingdom.

ANGER

Anger is the most destructive inner enemy both for ourselves and others. It is generated by feelings such as envy, jealousy, pride, selfishness and a mental attitude which states 'I am right and you are wrong'. A person who is angry has no patience and no time to think clearly what it is they want to do, they will try instead to do everything on the spot. This can often lead to misfortune and failure. When this happens they will blame others for their mistakes and they might even become abusive and physically violent, leading to further actions which harm and kill.

When we are angry it feels like the anger is coming from the middle of our body around the region of our liver and gall bladder. In English we say when we are angry, 'My blood is boiling'. It changes the colour of our face and increases our bodily temperature. Constant anger can disrupt our heat energy and cause disorders related to *mKhris-pa*. Anger is symbolized in the medical texts by a snake. It is helpful when you feel angry to visualize yourself standing in front of a snow-capped mountain which is able to melt the fire-like anger. It is also helpful to visualize how ugly anger can be, by picturing someone whose face is distorted by it. And if, for example, we have feelings of anger towards our parents we should visualize them as old, grey and full of wrinkles; how can we then feel angry towards those who are obviously no threat to us ?

DELUSION

Delusion is like a fog which permeates our mind and body and generates laziness. Due to laziness we leave everything to the last minute, we do not want to do much physical activity like exercise or cooking proper food, and sometimes we do not even want to think. Because of this we wish to do everything in the easiest, cheapest and quickest way. This behaviour can lead to us becoming overweight and mentally dull, which in turn disrupts our bodily fluids and causes *Bad-Kan* disorders.

SHORT-TERM CAUSES

These are:

1 Improper diet and lifestyle
2 Seasonal factors
3 Spirits

1) IMPROPER DIET AND LIFESTYLE

In the West scientists are still investigating whether there is a connection between illness and diet. However in Tibetan medicine it has already been confirmed that improper diet and lifestyle can cause physical and mental illnesses. From my experience of three different kinds of society – Tibetan, Indian and Western – I can say that different countries have different illnesses connected with their people's eating habits and the way the people lead their lives.

In the Tibetan community people drink butter tea (a combination of butter, salt, milk and tea churned together) in excessive amounts, much more for example, than the amounts of tea which the English drink. As refugees the generation to which my parents belong have led strenuous physical lives. They performed work such as quarrying, demolishing rocks through the use of explosives, and road construction in North India; all these in extreme climates of heat and cold. Therefore the biggest problems within the elder Tibetan community are hypertension (which is caused through taking in too much salt), arthritis, and eye, hearing and back problems (caused by a life of physical hardship).

By contrast to the Tibetans, Indians love sweets and hot spicy foods. They drink too much iced water in the summer months, chew too much *pan* (a mixture of beetle leaf, beetle nut, slaked lime and other herbs and spices) and they smoke too many *beedis* (a very popular cheap Indian cigarette). In the large cities – where the populations are huge – there are not many facilities for them to engage in physical exercise, therefore Indian people are often unfit. Due to these factors the main health problems in India are diabetes, asthma, ulcers, mouth and throat cancer and obesity.

In the West people eat too much sugar in the form of sweets, chocolate and fizzy drinks, and consume too much fatty and starchy foods. They also drink too much tea, coffee and alcohol and smoke too much. The lifestyle is generally very fast with people constantly rushing around and having little time to relax. In the cities the majority of people are employed in jobs which involve sitting at a desk and therefore they do not do too much physical exercise. Many people also drive to work and can therefore quite easily spend their working day doing very little walking at all. These factors lead to problems such as heart disease, cancer, insomnia, depression, tooth decay, digestive disorders, skin and weight problems. These examples illustrate the link between improper diet and unwholesome lifestyle and mental and physical illnesses.

CAUSES AND CONDITIONS WHICH IMBALANCE THE NYES-PA-GSUM.

We have already discussed the type, location and function of *Loong, mKhris-pa* and *Bad-Kan* within the body; here we will see the effects of them being disrupted.

Loong is one of the three principal energies of the body and has the nature of the air element. It is characterized by being movable, light, cold, subtle, hard and rough. The subtle flow of *Loong* is disrupted if we take in excess food and drink which have the same characteristics as *Loong*. These are coffee, tea, pork, goat's milk, yoghurt, white and black peppers, white bread, coca cola, chocolate, grapefruit, lemon and lime. *Loong* is disrupted when we perform actions such as fasting and giving ourselves too much mental stress, suffer excess blood loss from the body either through accident or labour, have too much sexual activity, skip meals or do not eat at the appropriate times. The natural flow of *Loong* will also be disrupted if we suffer from chronic diarrhoea and vomiting, grieve too much for loved ones we have lost, talk excessively, try to repress the normal eliminating functions of the body, physically strain ourselves too much on an empty stomach, cry until we collapse and work long hours without rest.

mKhris-pa has the same nature as the fire element. It is characterized by being hot, sharp, oily, of strong odour, purgative and fluid. Our bodily heat is increased and *mKhris-pa* is disrupted if we take in excess food and drink with similar characteristics to it, such as alcohol (especially spirits like whisky), lamb, duck, eggs, garlic, chilli, butter, milk, full fat cheese and cream, nuts and seeds. Wrong actions such as doing too much strenuous physical exercise in the heat, constantly being full of anger, sleeping in the middle of the day, doing excess physical labour such as digging when gardening, can also lead to *mKhris-pa* disorders.

Bad-Kan has the same nature as the water and earth elements. The characteristics of *Bad-Kan* are heavy, smooth, blunt, oily, cool, firm and sticky. *Bad-Kan* energy is disrupted if we take in excess food and drink with the same characteristics as it, such as sugar, potatoes, raw milk, raw vegetables, cold foods, half-cooked meats and chilled drinks. Wrong actions such as sleeping on a full stomach, eating late at night, eating too fast, exposing our bodies to cold weather by wearing inadequate clothing, eating before the food eaten previously has been properly digested and not performing enough physical exercise can all lead to *Bad-Kan* disorders such as indigestion and water retention.

Loong and *Bad-Kan* disorders are very common in the West while *mKhris-pa* disorders are common in countries which have a hot climate, such as India.

ILLNESSES CAUSED THROUGH MISUSE OF THE FIVE SENSES

The five senses can become damaged through over-use. For example, the eyes can become strained from sitting in front of a computer screen for hours and hours, watching too much television, reading continuously, or focusing on an object which is either too big or too small. If you sit in a dark place which has no natural light eye problems can also occur. In some cases the visual effect from seeing something repulsive such as vomit, faeces or blood can cause people to be sick and in some cases illness can be caused merely by seeing something such as a snake slithering in the grass. These examples give some indication of the power of the sense of sight.

ILLNESSES CAUSED THROUGH MISUSE OF MIND, BODY AND SPEECH

The body can be strained by physical activities, and in professions such as nursing and gardening, the most common problems are back related (due to lifting patients and digging the ground). Varicose veins can be a problem for people whose work involves a lot of standing. Physical strains can also occur in jobs which require less heavy labour. For example, repetitive strain injury through typing.

Recently I saw a female patient in her late forties who is a real-estate agent and who spends many hours on the telephone talking to clients. As a result her neck was bent towards the right and, due to it being stiff, she was unable to straighten it. I prescribed herbal medicines to relax the muscles and nerves in her neck and on a practical level I advised her to buy a telephone with headphones so that this problem would not reoccur.

Another case is a patient of mine who is in his early forties and who does a lot of computer work as a book editor. He strained his wrist and arm to such an extent that he had to take a long rest from his work in order to recover. This shows how repetitive actions can lead to physical strains. In the same way if we do very little physical activity problems may occur, such as gaining too much weight, obesity and listlessness.

The mind can be strained by such things as continually focusing on one subject, worrying over something such as money, the possibility of losing a job or a partner, grieving for a loved one, being consumed by desire for promotion at work, or even worrying about one's age. All these factors can contribute to complaints such as high blood pressure, heart disease and insomnia.

When the mind is underused, it can forget what it knows. In my own case, when I was working at the Tibetan Medical and Astrological Institute branch clinic in New Delhi I had to learn Hindi in order to be able to communicate with the mainly Indian patients. During that time I was able to speak Hindi quite well and I was able to use the relevant medical terms. However, since being in England for some years, where I have no need to speak Hindi, I have forgotten a great deal of this.

Speech can be strained by activities such as continually shouting, screaming and even singing. To a lesser extent people in professions such as teaching, lecturing, politics and entertainment can get very exhausted through having to talk all day. It can also be the case that when some people talk continually even the people listening to them can become exhausted! From all these examples we can see it is important to be moderate in our use of the five senses and our body, speech and mind.

2) SEASONAL FACTORS

The Tibetan lunar calendar is divided into six seasons – late winter, spring, dry summer, wet summer, autumn and early winter. It is very important for each season to occur at the right time, otherwise when it is too hot, too wet or too cold the external imbalance of the season will lead to internal imbalance of the three principal energies of *Loong*, *mKhris-pa* and *Bad-Kan*.

During the dry summer, which in the American and European calendar corresponds to the months May and June, the environmental qualities become light and dry. These have the same characteristics as *Loong*. Therefore if you are *Loong* in nature and if you eat lots of non-nutritious light and rough food, along with having mental stress, *Loong* will *accumulate* in your body.

During the wet summer – which corresponds to July and August – the environment becomes cooler due to rain and wind. This aggravates *Loong* and it becomes *manifest*, leading to illness. This is shown by the fact that breathing problems such as asthma, bronchitis and joint problems worsen during this time.

During autumn – which corresponds to September and October – the environment qualities become warm and oily, they counteract and *pacify Loong*.

For *mKhris-pa* during wet summer (July and August) the environmental qualities become cool and oily. If you are *mKhris-pa* in nature and you eat lots of hot, sharp and sour potency food and you perform lots of strenuous physical activity, *mKhris-pa accumulates* in the body.

In the autumn (September and October) the environmental qualities become warm and oily which aggravates *mKhris-pa* and therefore *mKhris-pa* disorders become *manifest*. This leads to illnesses such as headaches, high blood pressure and the flaring up of skin diseases.

In early winter – which corresponds to November and December – the environmental qualities become cold which counteract and *pacify mKhris-pa*.

In late winter – which corresponds to January and February – the environmental qualities are cold, heavy, blunt and oily. If your body nature is *Bad-Kan* and you eat lots of cold and raw food and do little exercise, *Bad-Kan accumulates*.

In the spring – which corresponds to March and April – the environmental qualities are warm and *Bad-Kan* disorders *manifest* causing digestive problems, asthma, colds, flu and weight problems.

In the dry summer (May and June) the environmental qualities become light and dry which counteract the *Bad-Kan* and *pacify* it.

3) INFLUENCE OF SPIRITS

Tibetans believe in the influence of spirits. When a Tibetan physician treats a patient and there is no response, despite the diagnosis and treatment being correct, it will be due to the influence of spirits. The physician will therefore recommend that the patient sees a recognized spiritual practitioner. The spirits will then be exorcised from the patient through performing rituals such as cake offerings, fire pujas, mantra recitations and reading holy Buddhist scriptures such as the Tibetan *Kangyur* and *Tengyur*.

The influence of spirits can be caused by frequent engagement of non-meritorious deeds such as killing other sentient beings, breaking religious precepts by not performing offerings and commitments, destroying images of spirits and making disparaging remarks about them, engaging excessively in non-productive verbal and physical activities, being tormented by continuous mental suffering and finally by living in isolation with no contact with other people. There are 18 different types of spirits listed in the Tibetan medical texts which can possess people and manifest themselves through physical symptoms.

Table Showing the Relationship Between Disease and Seasonal Factors

Tibetan Month	European/ US Month	Seasons	Environmental Qualities	Accumulation in the Body	Manifestation of Disorder	Pacification of Imbalance
12, 1	1, 2	Late Winter	Cold, heavy, oily	*Bad-Kan*		
2, 3	3, 4	Spring	Warm		*Bad-Khan*	
4, 5	5, 6	Dry Summer	Light, dry	*Loong*		*Bad-Khan*
6, 7	7, 8	Wet Summer	Oily, cool	*MKhris-pa*	*Loong*	
8, 9	9, 10	Autumn	Warm, oily		*MKhris-pa*	*Loong*
10, 11	11, 12	Early Winter	Cold			*MKhris-pa*

1 Desire realm gods spirits. Symptoms of the patient being possessed by this spirit are an obsession with cleanliness (such as the repeated washing of hands), always favouring the colour white in their choice of clothing, speaking in an unknown language, loss of appetite.
2 Semi-God realm spirits. Symptoms are a fondness for eating meat and drinking alcohol, violent and stubborn behaviour, non-stop talking, no direct eye contact with people and always looking out of the corner of their eyes.
3 Scent eating spirits. The symptoms of the patient are an obsession with appearance such as the frequent changing of their clothes, a fondness for perfumes and music, a preference for the colour red.
4 *Naga* or water spirits. The symptoms of the patient are staring red eyes, a love of meat and milk, excessive thirst, constant licking of the mouth and dripping of saliva, always sleeping on their stomach and never on their back or side.
5 Mountain spirits. The symptoms of the patient are excessive generosity, whispered speech, walking in a hurry, a dislike of doctors, a fondness for fish.
6 Brahma spirits. The symptoms of the patient are a constant calling out to people, pretending to read books or scriptures, physically hurting themselves and frightening others with weapons, laughing loudly and continuously.
7 Cannibal ogre spirits. The symptoms of the patient are abusive verbal behaviour, excess physical strength, a love of red meat, clothes, jewellery and flowers, crying, loss of interest in cleanliness, collapsing and loss of consciousness, wandering at night.
8 Flesh eating spirits. The symptoms of the patient are excessive feelings of shyness and guilt, tantrums, constant hunger, a fondness for horse riding and climbing trees.

9 Hungry ghost spirits. The symptoms of the patient are that they become very thin, especially their limbs, very frightened and nervous, they become suspicious and nosy, they no longer have any appetite for food which they previously adored.

10 Jug shaped spirits. Symptoms are a very serious facial expression, walking at an extremely slow pace, swollen scrotum which hangs.

11 Curse caused spirits. The symptoms of the patient are they always carry soil or wood in their hands, running naked, becoming abusive.

12 Distracting spirits. The symptoms of the patient are always drinking water, always complaining, possessing no appetite.

13 Zombie spirits. The symptoms of the patient are an obsession with sleep, an insistence that whatever they say is the truth, constant shivering.

14 Ancestral spirits. This spirit can enter into one of the remaining members of the family of a deceased person and act and talk like the deceased. The patient's mouth is always dry and they cannot bear the light and always want to close their eyes. The unique characteristic of this spirit is that the possessed person will always wear their clothes from the left side.

15 Teacher spirits.

16 Hermit spirits

17 God physician spirits

18 Tantrician spirits.

These final four types of spirit are mainly the creation of black magicians and their purpose is to harm others. They are very difficult to cure, unlike the rest of the above which can be successfully treated.

One example I have relates to the Curse caused spirit. When I was growing up in the Tibetan refugee community of Bylakuppe in South India, there was an incident involving a recently married young woman in our village. People said that she had been cursed by her mother-in-law and had become possessed. She would walk with a stick in her hand and run naked throughout the village. The community invited a famous and highly respected local tantric practitioner called Chakham Tulku. He performed a fire puja to exorcize the spirit and successfully cured the young woman. To this day you can still see the scars on her arms as a result of her jumping into the flames during the fire ritual.

All of the above 18 different types of spirits can enter our consciousness and transform our physical gestures, the way we speak and our mental thinking. They can make the patient unfocused, restless, quick-tempered and confused.

Once the three principal energies are unbalanced we become unhealthy and are in a diseased state.

HOW DISEASE ENTERS THE BODY

GENERAL PATHWAYS OF DISEASE

1 Skin – in the beginning the disease spreads on the skin.
2 Muscle tissues – disease develops in the muscle tissues.
3 Vessels – moves through the blood vessels and nerves.
4 Bones – affects the bones and marrow.
5 Five vital organs – disease advances to the heart, liver, lungs, spleen and kidneys.
6 Six hollow organs – descends into the stomach, small intestine, gall bladder, urinary bladder, large intestine, reproductive organs.

SPECIFIC PATHWAYS OF DISEASE

1 *Loong* moves through the bones, ears, skin, heart, blood vessels, nerves and large intestine.
2 *mKhris-pa* moves through the blood, eyes, sweat, liver, gall bladder and small intestine.
3 *Bad-Kan* moves through essential nutrients, muscle tissue, fat, marrow, regenerative fluids, the nose and tongue, lower bodily passages connected with urination and defecation, lungs, spleen, kidneys and urinary bladder.

Once disease has entered our body, there are three factors to be considered and they are related to age, place and time.

FACTORS RELATING TO AGE

- Aged person. Here the overall bodily energy is diminished because of the ageing process and this can make the person susceptible to *Loong* disorders. Because of this, when we get older we need less sleep.
- Adult person. Here the overall bodily energy should be at its peak and this can make the person susceptible to hot *mKhris-pa* disorders. Because of this, when we are young we are full of courage and determination.
- Young person. Children have an overall bodily energy which is sensitive and still developing, and they are susceptible to *Bad-Kan* disorders. Because of this, children need lots of sleep.

FACTORS RELATING TO PLACE

- *Loong* develops and accumulates in cold and windy regions.
- *MKhris-pa* develops and accumulates in hot and dry regions
- *Bad-Kan* develops and accumulates in damp and humid regions.

FACTORS RELATED TO TIME

- *Loong* disorders manifest during the summer, evening and dawn. It is because of this that *Loong* medicine is prescribed to be taken in the morning and in the evening.
- *mKhris-pa* disorders manifest during autumn, midnight and midday. It is because of this that *mKhris-pa* medicine is prescribed to be taken either at midday or at midnight.
- *Bad-Kan* disorders manifest in the spring, dusk and morning. It is because of this that *Bad-Kan* medicine is prescribed to be taken in the morning and evening.

MANIFESTATION OF DISEASE

Once the three *Nyes-pas*, the seven bodily constituents and the three eliminating functions are either in excess in our body, or are deficient and disrupted, we will see the following signs and symptoms of sickness:

EXCESS, DEFICIENCY AND DISRUPTION OF LOONG, mKhris-pa AND BAD-KAN

EXCESS OF LOONG

- Weight loss, constipation, flatulence, insomnia, dizziness, tiredness, dark complexion, always feeling cold, weakening of eyesight.

LOONG DEFICIENCY

- Forgetfulness, fatigue, withdrawal, aches and pains throughout the body.

DISRUPTION OF LOONG

- The pulse when read by the physician is empty and floating, the urine is light and clear with big bubbles. There will be constant sighing, restlessness, unfocussed mind and loss of physical balance, ringing in the ears, unlocalized shifting pain, stiffness and contraction in the limbs, pain in the eyeballs, sensitive skin, dryness on the tongue, astringent taste, shivering and feeling feverish, pain in the joints when the slightest movement is made, sleeplessness, constant yawning, constant desire to stretch, irritability, pain in the back and hip joints, sensation of vomiting when there is nothing to be vomited, a frothy mucus coming out of the mouth in the dawn and evening. When the physician presses the selected points of *Loong*, such as the temples, the first, fifth and sixth vertebrae and the sternum, they become very sensitive and painful; discomfort is especially felt in the dawn and early evening.

EXCESS OF mKhris-pa

- The colour of the skin, sclera, stools and urine turns yellow, there is excess hunger and thirst, high temperature, diarrhoea and very little sleep.

mKhris-pa DEFICIENCY

- There is loss of bodily heat, the hands and feet become cold, and there is a darkening of complexion.

DISRUPTION OF mKhris-pa

- The pulse when read by the physician is thin, twisted and fast, and the urine is a yellowish-red colour with a strong odour and vapour. There will be headaches, high temperature, sour and bitter taste on the tongue and it will have a thick pale yellow coating, uncontrollable sleep in the daytime but an inability to sleep at night, yellowing of sclera, excruciating pain in the liver and gall bladder, sputum will become salty and sour, feeling of sickness due to bile, diarrhoea, perspiration and sweat will have a very bad odour and skin complexion becomes very yellow; discomfort is especially felt in the daytime and at midnight and when digesting food.

EXCESS OF BAD-KAN

- Indigestion, feeling of heaviness in the body, excess mucus and saliva, pale complexion, lifeless feeling of the limbs, difficulty in breathing, uncontrollable sleep, laziness and apathy.

BAD-KAN DEFICIENCY

- There is no strength due to poor absorption, dizziness, palpitations, the joints become floppy.

DISRUPTION OF BAD-KAN

- The pulse when read by the physician is slow and weak, and the urine is whitish in colour with no odour and vapour. There is a loss of taste, the tongue, gums and sclera become pale, puffiness of the face, disorientation of the mind and heaviness in the body, loss of appetite, poor absorption, constant clearing of the throat due to excess mucus formation, pain in the kidneys and back, water retention, loss of memory, excess weight gain, apathy, feelings of discomfort after eating, and feelings of discomfort especially at dawn and dusk and when it is damp.

EXCESS AND DEFICIENCY OF THE SEVEN BODILY CONSTITUENTS

ESSENTIAL NUTRIENTS

- When in excess, the rate of metabolism is reduced and there is difficulty in digesting food. When deficient there is loss of weight, difficulty in swallowing food, the skin becomes dry and rough, there is a throbbing sound in the ears and aches and pains all over the body.

BLOOD

- When in excess there are skin problems, tumours, jaundice, gum disease, hypertension, bloodshot eyes, leprosy, spleen disease. When deficient there is tiredness, dry skin, constant feeling of cold.

MUSCLE TISSUES

- When in excess there is goitre, weight increase, glandular diseases. When deficient there is excruciating pain in all the joints as if they are about to break, the skeleton is visible as there are just bones and skin with no muscle.

FATTY TISSUE

- When in excess there is heaviness in the body and mind, the breasts and stomach increase in size. When deficient there is lack of sleep, loss of weight and pale skin.

BONES

- When in excess there is extra bone and teeth growth. When deficient the hair, nails and teeth fall out.

BONE MARROW

- When in excess eyesight becomes weaker, joints become enlarged, the whole body becomes sensitive. When deficient bones become brittle, there is giddiness and there are cataracts in the eyes.

REGENERATIVE FLUID (SPERM)

- When in excess there is a very high sex drive and a constant desire for a sexual partner. If not released, excess sperm might lead to urinary and kidney stones. When deficient through over-use, there is bleeding and painful burning sensations.

EXCESS AND DEFICIENCY OF THE THREE ELIMINATING FUNCTIONS

FAECES

- When in excess it causes heaviness in the body, a bloated stomach, intestinal pain and rumbling in the stomach. When deficient it causes chronic diarrhoea. The intestines are full of gas which can sometimes move upwards and cause pain in the heart and the ribs.

URINE

- When in excess there is pain for men when urinating and a frequent desire to urinate (even when just recently urinated). When deficient there is very little urine, it is very difficult to release and becomes very concentrated.

PERSPIRATION

- When in excess there is lots of sweating, strong body odour, itchiness and other skin problems. When deficient the skin becomes chapped and cracked and there is loss of body hair.

5

HUMAN ANATOMY AND PHYSIOLOGY

HUMAN EMBRYOLOGY

In the Tibetan medical texts the formation of the human body is divided into:

1 Human conception
2 Development
3 Childbirth

1) HUMAN CONCEPTION

Human conception is divided into primary and secondary causes. Although we think human birth is easy and is often something we take for granted, according to both the Tibetan medical and Tibetan Buddhist conceptual systems, to get the human form is as rare and precious as a daytime star.

The **primary** causes of human birth are the father's sperm and the mother's ovum. The sperm and ovum should be absolutely free from the nine defects that are mentioned in the Tibetan medical texts:

1 If there is *Loong* disorder the semen and menstrual blood are very coarse and black in colour.

2 If there is *mKhris-pa* disorder the semen and menstrual blood are yellowish and have a strong odour.
3 If there is *Bad-Kan* disorder the semen and menstrual blood are very pale and sticky.
4 If there is a blood disorder the semen and menstrual blood are rotten and mushy.
5 If it is a combination of *Bad-Kan* and *Loong* disorders the semen and menstrual blood are in pieces.
6 If it is a combination of blood and *mKhris-pa* disorders the semen and menstrual blood are like pus and very cloudy.
7 If it is a combination of *Bad-Kan* and *mKhris-pa* the semen and menstrual blood are clotted.
8 If it is a combination of *Loong* and *mKhris-pa* the flow of the menstrual cycle stops and if there happens to be any, it is very little.
9 If is a multiple combination of *Loong, mKhris-pa, Bad-Kan* and blood disorders, the semen and menstrual blood are solid like faeces.

The last two defects are difficult to treat but all the rest are treatable.

Therefore for healthy conception the semen and ovum must be healthy. Healthy semen should be white in colour, thick, plentiful, sweet in taste, and overall the texture should be like honey. The menstrual blood should be red like rabbits' blood and if it stains it can easily be washed.

The semen of the father generates the bone, brain and spinal cord. The mother's ovum generates muscle tissue, the five vital organs (heart, lungs, liver, spleen, kidneys) and the six hollow organs (stomach, small intestine, large intestine, gall bladder, urinary bladder, reproductive organs). It is the consciousness – *nam-shey* – which generates the five senses of sight, taste, smell, hearing and touch.

The final primary cause of human conception is the *nam-shey*, or consciousness, which is wandering without form in the *Bardo* (intermediate state between life and death) looking for its karmic parents through which to take rebirth. In the Tibetan Buddhist scripture called *Do-dhe Kunchok Tsekpa* the Buddha instructed his disciple *Kungawo* that to get the human body we need both causes and conditions for the connection between the wandering consciousness and its future parents. Sometimes there is the cause but no conditions, such as the parents being there but both of them having no mood for sexual intercourse, or they are ill at the time and therefore unable to do so.

Similarly the parents are there and are sexually active but they themselves are of high birth and have accumulated much spiritual merit, while the consciousness trying to take rebirth has little, and is therefore incompatible. It might be the case that both parents and consciousness are equal but the time is not right; this is one of the reasons why some couples have to wait a long time to bear a child. In Tibetan society if a couple have not conceived after a long time they would be advised to do lots of spiritual practice and purification rituals in order to accumulate merit and thus create the conditions for conception.

The **secondary** causes of childbirth are the five elements. Earth elements help the foetus to be solid, water elements give it cohesion, fire elements mature the foetus, air elements aid growth and development and finally space elements help the foetus to move.

If there is earth but no water element, it is like flour which without water cannot be formed into dough. If there is water but no earth element the water will flow and not remain in one place. If there is earth and water but no fire element it is like in the middle of the summer when an animal carcass is left in the shade without any sun and it rots and decomposes. If there is earth, water and fire but no air elements it is like making bread when we have to knead the dough slowly in order for the air to circulate and the dough itself to rise and expand. If there is earth, water, fire and air but no space elements it is like trying to fit your feet into shoes which are too small and your feet get painful and squashed.

Earth generates the solid substances in our body such as bones, muscle tissue, the nose and the sense of smell. Water generates the fluid substances in our body such as blood and other bodily fluids, the tongue and its sense of taste. Fire generates bodily heat, clarity of complexion, the eyes and their sense of sight. Air generates breath as well as the skin and the sense of touch. Space generates the various orifices, the ears and their sense of hearing. The sperm and ovum are produced from all the five elements.

The embryo is thus formed by having healthy semen and ovum, consciousness, and the five elements.

2) DEVELOPMENT

The development of the foetus takes 38 weeks and this is divided into three stages.

The first stage is called the fish stage of development (weeks one to nine) and at this stage the foetus is fish-shaped with no visible limbs. This stage is the most vulnerable stage for the development of the foetus and during it the mother should be especially careful about her diet and conduct. She should avoid strenuous physical exertion such as lifting heavy objects, vigorous sexual intercourse, going to sleep late at night or sleeping in the daytime. It is important that she should relax mentally. With regard to diet, if it is possible she should avoid alcohol, strong medication, smoking, chillis and fish. The reason for having to avoid fish is because it is able to dissolve tumours and therefore it might also dissolve the foetus when it is in its formative stages.

If possible the mother should eat organic food such as fresh vegetables, fresh fruit, pulses, rice, lean beef, free range chicken and eggs, organic milk and yoghurt and cereals. If the mother does not take care of her diet and conduct during this time there is the possibility of miscarriage. Whatever the mother eats or drinks is absorbed by her digestive system and its essence is stored in her reproductive organs, and these are connected to the two channels of the uterus by the umbilical cord which in turn develops the foetus.

The second stage of development is called the turtle stage of development (weeks 10 to 17) and at this stage the shape of the foetus is like a turtle. The limbs have appeared, as have the five vital organs, the six hollow organs, the six senses and the connective nerves and channels. Now it is safe for the mother to eat fish.

The third stage of development is called the pig stage of development (weeks 18 to 35) and at this stage everything is developed and functional. It is called the pig stage as the foetus is now conscious of its surroundings. From week 24 the senses of the foetus are fully functioning and from this time the mother should avoid very hot drinks, chilli, alcohol and smoking.

Weeks 36, 37 and 38 are the preparation stages for delivery and during these final stages there are signs and symptoms as to whether the baby will be a boy or a girl. If it is a boy, the right side of the mother's abdomen is higher than the left and milk starts dripping from her right breast; her dreams will be of men and in her dreams she will have strong sexual desire. If it is a girl the left side of the mother's abdomen is higher than the right and milks drips from her left breast, her dreams will be of flowers, jewellery and in her dreams she will especially feel like listening to songs and music. If it is twins both the left and right sides of the abdomen are high and the middle is a little hollow.

3) CHILDBIRTH

The majority of women have no problems when they are delivering; however there are three obstacles to an easy birth. Firstly, if the mother has heavy internal bleeding which can prevent the growth of the foetus, the baby will be stillborn. Secondly, if the mother has put on a great deal of weight during pregnancy the vaginal canals will be blocked and the foetus will be unable to come out, resulting in a caesarean birth. Thirdly, due to improper diet and conduct the downward cleansing *Loong* moves upward and causes delay in the delivery. Generally it is important for the mother to take a daily walk and try to mentally relax in order to avoid the problems mentioned above.

The skin of a new born baby is very sensitive and delicate, therefore it is highly advisable to wrap it in smooth fabric such as silk. When bathing the baby it is very important that the water is exactly at the right temperature, being neither too hot – or too cold. There is a vast difference between the sensitivity of the skin of our fingers – which we use to check the water temperature – and the skin of a new born baby. If the water is too hot, the baby feels like it is being put in melted iron, and if it is too cold it feels like it is being put in ice.

At this time full attention should also be given to the mother, as the mother's diet is crucial for the wellbeing and future healthy growth of the child. The mother should try to eat as much organic food as possible, if this is not possible she should at least eat a lot of fresh fruit and vegetables. She should avoid all kinds of processed food and food which contains artificial additives. Finally the mother should feed the baby with her milk for at least a year, with lots of love.

THE ORGANS

This section looks at the five vital organs, the six hollow organs and metaphors for the human body.

As in the other medical sciences, in Tibetan medicine there are five vital and six hollow organs. It is very important for the physician to know the exact location of these organs in order to perform external therapies such as blood-letting and moxibustion and to find internal disorders.

Compared to other oriental medicines Tibetan medical knowledge of the internal anatomy of the body is quite extensive. Due to cultural reasons to open the body in many Asian countries is seen as a sign of disrespect, though this has never been the case in Tibet. This is illustrated by the traditional Tibetan method of sky burial where the body is cut open into pieces and left for the wild birds. In the course of Tibetan medical history, one of Tibet's most well-known physicians, Dhak-po Menrampa, on the death of his mother, dissected her body and found that her stomach had shrunk. This was due to the chronic digestive disorders from which she suffered and therefore he was able to make a new medicine called *Dhak-Men 15* which contains 15 ingredients to help chronic digestive problems and which is still in use today.

When checking the exact location of the organs the physician places the patient on a flat mattress. The patient sits cross-legged with their back being as straight as an arrow, their head is bent slightly forward, their shoulders are pushed back and their hands are resting on their knees.

FIVE VITAL ORGANS

The upper trunk consists of the lungs and heart. In Tibetan medical anatomy the lungs are divided into the five posterior lobes and the five interior lobes. The posterior lobes are known in Tibetan as the mother lungs and they are situated at the back. The interior lobes are known as the son lungs and they are situated in the front. The heart sits on top of the posterior lobes like a king on his throne.

The lower trunk contains the remaining three vital organs. The liver on the right side is compared to a rock sitting on a precipice and pointing upwards. The spleen is thinner in the middle and thicker at the outer edges, it is located just below the stomach. The left and right kidneys are in an upright position and are compared to bodyguards.

SIX HOLLOW ORGANS

Of the six hollow organs the stomach is the storage space for ingested food, its shape is wider in the upper part and narrower in the lower part. The small intestine connected to the stomach is like a gutter filled with water. The large intestine is connected to the small intestine and is divided into three sections, the ascending, transverse and descending colons; the sigmoid colon and the rectum are also connected to the large intestine. The gall bladder is connected to the liver and looks like a pouch. The urinary bladder is like a storage jar. The reproductive organs are shaped like glands.

METAPHORS OF THE HUMAN BODY

In the Tibetan medical texts, metaphors were used to educate the lay people in an understanding of the physical anatomy.

The physical body – visualized sitting cross-legged, with a straight back and arms resting gently on the knees – is compared to a palace of a universal emperor. The walls of the palace foundation are like our hipbones, the vertebrae are like a stack of gold coins, the palace beams are like our ribs, and our flesh and skin is like the plaster of the building. The head is like a palace turret and the palace windows are like our five sense organs. The upper and lower parts of the trunk are like the upper and lower courtyards of the palace.

The five organs are described in order of their importance. The heart is like a king sitting on a throne, it is the most important organ in our body. The lungs are like the king's ministers, the liver and spleen are like the senior and junior queens and the kidneys are the king's foreign ministers.

Of the six hollow organs, the stomach is like a cooking pot, the small intestine and large intestine are like a queen's housemaids, the gall bladder is like a sack full of spices, the urinary bladder is like a water jar and the two lower passages of the anus and urethra are like two drainage gutters. Finally the legs are like arched pediments above the palace gates.

BONES

In Tibetan medicine there are 23 different classifications for bones.

- For the cranial bones there are five groups: the skull, occipital bones, nasal bones, teeth, mandible.
- For the trunk there are nine groups: vertebrae, vertebrae prominens, coccyx, hip bones, shoulder bones, collarbones, sternum, ribs, costal cartilages.
- For the arms there are three groups: humerus, forearm including the radius and ulna, the hand including carpals, metacarpals, phalanges.
- For the legs there are five groups: femur, lower leg including tibia and fibula, patella, calcaneus, the foot including the tarsals, metatarsals, phalanges.
- Finally there is a single group comprising of fingernails and toenails.

All the above bones are connected together by 12 major joints and 210 minor joints.

CHANNELS

There are four different types of channels (*rtsa*) in Tibetan medicine:

1 Embryonic formation channels
2 Existent channels
3 Connecting channels
4 Life force channels

When the channels intertwine nerve plexus are formed.

1) EMBRYONIC CHANNELS

The embryonic formation channels extend from the navel and divide into three sub-channels.

The first sub-channel extends upwards to form the brain. The brain is the source of all our thoughts and also the source of our ignorance as it is like an ocean of nerves. When we feel confused and heavy the feeling begins in our head. It is the location of *Bad-Kan* within our body.

The second sub-channel is the hepatic artery of the liver and this channel forms the black channel of life and the blood vessels. Blood is the cause of the heat which generates anger. This middle part of the body is the location of *mKhris-pa*.

The third sub-channel extends down to the genitalia plexus which is the source of pleasure and it is this channel which generates desire. *Loong* is located in the lower part of the body.

2) EXISTENT CHANNELS

The sensory organs are connected by 500 minor existent channels to the brain. For memory there are 500 minor existent channels connected to the heart plexus. The human body originates from the 500 minor channels in the navel plexus and offspring are produced in the 500 minor channels which originate in the genitalia plexus.

3) CONNECTING CHANNELS

All our channels are connected to each other throughout our body like a net. The connecting channels are divided into two: the black channel and the white channel.

The black channel, which means the arteries and veins in our body, is called the life channel because it sustains life. This channel originates from the liver, which is also the starting point of the 24 major blood vessels. The liver is vital for sustaining muscle tissue and blood. Eight of the 24 blood vessels are connected internally to the five vital and six hollow organs. There are then 16 external blood vessels connected with the limbs. In greater detail there are 77 blood-letting points and 112 vulnerable blood vessels which cannot be used for blood-letting as that would be fatal. In greater detail still, there are 360 minor blood vessels.

The white channel, or the nervous system, includes the brain, spinal cord and connected nerves. Its stem is located in the brain and it descends throughout our body. There are roughly 19 white channels:

- There are four white channels connected to the heart and small intestines and they help the functioning of *Loong*.
- There are four white channels connected to the lungs, large intestines, liver and gall bladder and they help the functioning of *mKhris-pa*.

- There are four white channels connected with the stomach, spleen, kidneys and urinary bladder and they help the functioning of *Bad-Kan*.
- There is one common white channel connected with the reproductive organs. There are six other channels connected externally such as two tubular channels, two precious channels and two paralytic channels. There are also 11 minor white channels.

4) LIFE FORCE CHANNELS

In Tibetan medicine life force energy is dependent on past karma and diet and behaviour followed in this life. There are three life force energies in our body which influence our life span:

- The first life force energy circulates throughout our body and this energy is the *medroy* or heat.

It is located in the stomach, intestines and colon as well as in the seven bodily constituents, especially the blood. This *medroy* gives us heat and protects us from cold and chills, it also gives us vitality and sustains our life. The *medroy* diminishes and degenerates as we get older. We can see for ourselves that as we become older our body temperature becomes colder, ending finally in death when our body becomes completely cold as the *medroy* has now been extinguished.

- The second life force energy circulates with the breath.
- The third life force energy is the *bla*, or *dhang*, which can be translated as meaning life essence.

Table showing monthly movement of bla (third life force) in a male body according to the Tibetan lunar calendar

Day	Location of bla	Day	Location of bla
1	Left big toe	16	Right cheek
2	Left ankle	17	Neck
3	Left calf	18	Right palm
4	Left knee	19	Right forearm
5	Back of left knee	20	Right shoulder
6	Left groin	21	Right ribs
7	Left hip	22	Right kidney
8	Left kidney	23	Right hip
9	Left ribs	24	Right groin
10	Left shoulder	25	Right back of knee
11	Left forearm	26	Right knee
12	Left palm	27	Right calf
13	Throat	28	Tarsals
14	Left cheek	29	Right ankle
15	Whole body	30	Whole body

This *bla* is located mainly in the heart, and it circulates from head to toe in a 30 day lunar cycle. In the male body the *bla* rotates from left to right, and in the female body it rotates from right to left. The physician has to know the exact whereabouts of the *bla* when performing therapies such as blood-letting and moxibustion. For example, on the first of the lunar calendar the *bla* moves in the big toe of a male body from left to right. During this time, if the physician wants to place moxa on this toe to treat a complaint such as swollen testicles, it is not advisable. How the *bla* rotates in full is shown in the table above.

VULNERABLE POINTS OF THE BODY

In Tibetan medicine the vulnerable points are divided into seven groups: vulnerable points of muscle tissue, fatty tissue, bone tissue, ligaments and tendons, vital and hollow viscera channels.

They are called vulnerable points when they are struck and damaged by weapons or through accidents. If muscle tissue is pulled or torn it swells up; if a bone is cracked or fractured there is unbearable pain; if the ligaments or tendons are damaged there is paralysis; if the nerves, fatty tissue or the vital and hollow organs are damaged it is life threatening.

For muscle tissue there are 45 vulnerable points:

- 5 vulnerable points in the head
- 4 in the neck
- 18 in the trunk
- 18 in the limbs

For fatty tissue there are 8 vulnerable points:

- 2 in the trunk
- 6 in the limbs

For bone tissue there are 32 vulnerable points:

- 14 on the head
- 5 in the neck
- 7 in the trunk
- 6 in the limbs

For ligaments and tendons there are 14 vulnerable points:

- 2 in the neck
- 2 in the trunk
- 10 in the limbs

For the vital and hollow viscera there are 13 vulnerable points:

- heart, lungs, liver, spleen, kidneys, stomach, gall bladder, small intestine, large intestine, urinary bladder, reproductive organs.

For the channels there 190 vulnerable points:

- 15 in the brain
- 14 in the bone channels
- 14 in muscle tissue
- 22 in the neck
- 53 in the trunk
- 72 in the limbs

In total there 322 vulnerable points in our body.

THE SEVEN BODILY NATURES

In Tibetan medical science, gender is divided into three: male, female and hermaphrodite. Age is also divided into three:

- from 1 to 16 is the child
- from 16 to 70 is the adult
- above 70 is the aged

In respect of the three *Nyes-pas* there are seven human types: *Loong* type, *mKhris-pa* type and *Bad-Kan* type. In addition, there are combinations of two types together: *Loong / mKhris-pa, Loong / Bad-Kan, mKhris-pa / Bad-Kan.* Finally, there is a combination of all three; *Loong, mKhris-pa* and *Bad-Kan.*

LOONG TYPES

From the three poisons of ignorance, anger and desire, *Loong* types are most closely associated with desire. This is symbolized by a bird which is seen as a very sexually active creature. The *Loong* type body frame is thin, short and stooped, their complexion is dark, their skin is dry and they do not like the cold and wind. They have a sensitive and fearful temperament, they are suspicious, they love songs and they laugh easily. Their metabolic rate is variable and they find it easy to lose weight but hard to gain it. Their joints crackle when they walk, they have a poor memory and they find it difficult to make decisions. They will suffer from constipation, they are poor sleepers and will age faster than normal as their skin will develop wrinkles very quickly. Their wealth will not be great and their life span is short.

mKHRIS-PA TYPES

mKhris-pa types are most closely associated with anger. This is symbolized by a snake which is seen as a very aggressive creature. Their body frame is medium and proportionate, complexion and hair colour slightly yellowish. Their temperament is hot, they are impatient, and they are proud, obsessive, jealous and intelligent. They have an intense metabolic rate and therefore their weight is always constant. Their bodily temperature is warm and slightly oily, they perspire a lot, have eye problems and male *mKhris-pa* types will become prematurely bald and grey. It is easy for *mKhris-pa* types to feel hungry and thirsty and they generally prefer a cool climate. They sleep easily and they can get up easily. Their wealth and life span are medium.

BAD-KAN TYPES

Bad-Kan types are most closely associated with ignorance. This is symbolized by the pig which is seen as a very ignorant animal. Their body frame is broad and of big build, their complexion is fair and oily, their temperament is patient and kind but they are very lazy. Their metabolic rate is sluggish and *Bad-Kan* types will suffer from obesity. Their bodily temperature is cold, their appetite is regular and they can resist hunger and thirst. Their eliminating functions are slow. They love sleep and find it difficult to get up. They do not age quickly. Their wealth and life span are long.

When you are looking for a partner it is important to know the temperament and physiology of the other person in order for you both to be compatible, and for the relationship to be harmonious. *Bad-Kan* and *Loong* types are good together, or *Bad-Kan* and *mKhris-pa*[4]. *Loong* and *Loong*, *mKhris-pa* and *mKhris-pa*, *Loong* and *mKhris-pa* and *Bad-Kan* and *Bad-Kan* should be avoided.

6

COMMON DISEASES AND ILLNESSES

In Tibetan medicine there are 404 diseases which are put into four main categories. These are:

1. 101 untreatable diseases caused by past karma.
2. 101 diseases caused by spirits which can be eliminated through exorcism, spiritual practices and rituals.
3. 101 diseases caused by improper diet and improper conduct in this life which can be cured by treatment. If these diseases are left untreated the patient will die.
4. 101 ostensible diseases which can be cured easily without any treatment.

The 101 diseases which arise through past karma manifest without any apparent cause. This can result in sudden death and they could be the result of actions inflicted by another person or by actions inflicted by oneself. We Tibetans, as Buddhists, believe that this could come about as a result of one's actions in a previous life, specifically non-virtuous actions such as harming or even killing other beings. Because of this belief, if a Tibetan family suffers such a misfortune they will try not to blame others and will try to understand it is the result of their own past actions.

To purify themselves and to avoid further misfortune and illness, Tibetans will go on pilgrimage to holy places which have been blessed by holy beings. There they will perform such spiritual practices as reciting mantras and doing prostrations. They will also try to accumulate positive spiritual merit by helping those less fortunate and performing acts such as offering food and clothing to monks and nuns. We can see from our experience that some people try all forms of treatment with the best doctors and facilities and still they cannot be helped. This is because of past karma and failure to purify themselves through good deeds.

The remaining 303 diseases can all be helped through proper diet and conduct, proper medication and through the performing of various spiritual practices. In this chapter some of the more common diseases found in this country are explained from the Tibetan medical point of view.

1 Cold
2 Heart disease
3 Arthritis
4 Respiratory diseases
5 Skin diseases
6 Diabetes
7 Poisons
8 Child care and childhood diseases
9 Gynaecological diseases

1) THE COMMON COLD

In Tibetan cold is called *champa* and it is divided into four sections: causative factors, types of *champa*, symptoms and treatment.

CAUSATIVE FACTORS

Causative factors of *champa* are when there is extreme weather, either too hot or too cold, which upsets the *mKhris-pa* energy (*mKhris-pa* is what regulates bodily temperature, see page 14) or when dust and pollution enter through the mouth and nasal cavities and cause colds.

TYPES OF CHAMPA

There are four types of *champa* such as cold related to the throat, cold related to the lungs and cold related to the nose. Finally there is cold related to flu.

SYMPTOMS OF CHAMPA

The symptoms of *champa* related to the throat are, firstly the throat palate and vocal cavity become sore, next the nose begins to run which affects the vocal chords and there can be the loss of voice, then there is continuous sneezing.

The symptoms of *champa* related to the lungs are similar to the symptoms related to the throat with the addition of coughing, headaches, pain and congestion in the chest. With this type of cold one needs to get immediate treatment, otherwise it could become chronic and lead to bronchitis and other lung related diseases.

The symptoms of *champa* related to the nose are itchy and inflamed nostrils, and constant dripping of mucus from the nose.

The symptoms of *champa* related to flu are headaches, pain and aches in all the joints, pain in the calves, stiffness in the neck and hips, loss of appetite, temperature and shivering, bitter taste in the mouth, extreme feelings of discomfort in the evenings as if you have been badly beaten, you might also suffer from hallucinations and unclear dreams. At this time it is important to rest, avoid exertion and avoid a high protein diet. It is also important to avoid alcohol which, if taken, will increase the bodily temperature, burn the bodily system and in some cases even lead to death.

TREATMENT

In the beginning a decoction (the essence from extracting the water-soluble substances from a plant by boiling) is given which is called *Elecampane 4* – or seven precious decoctions – the main ingredient of which is emblica officinalis (one fruit of which contains as much vitamin C as two dozen oranges). These decoctions will help to balance the bodily temperature and build up the immune system. We can also prescribe medicines such as *Clove 6* for the throat, *Gentiana 15* for the lungs and *Camphor 25* for flu. For flu it is best to drink plenty of hot water and fast.

2) HEART DISEASE

According to Tibetan medicine the heart is the seat of the mind. The all pervasive *Loong* helps the heart to pump and circulate blood throughout our body. When we are frightened we can see the close connection between the heart and mind as it is the heart which jumps and not other organs such as our liver or kidneys. This description of the various types of heart disease is taken from the thirty-fourth chapter of the third Tibetan medical tantra. In Tibetan this chapter is called *nying ne* or heart disease. It is divided into four: causative factors of heart disease, types, symptoms and treatment.

CAUSATIVE FACTORS

In the Tibetan medical texts it is stated that every illness has a cause, if there were no cause how would it be possible to treat the disease? The causative factors of heart disease are, for example, mental stress caused by our own mind which is full of desire, selfishness, ambition and competitiveness. These emotions can put a great deal of strain on the subtle flow of the all pervasive *Loong* (which, when healthy, helps the circulation and pumping of blood throughout our body, see page 11).

We can strain our heart many times each day without being aware of what we are doing. This is especially true for people in highly paid professions where there can be great pressure on them, such as meeting deadlines, gaining new business and increasing profits for the company, and generally trying to do too much in order to gain promotion.

This lifestyle can mean that people do not look after themselves in ways such as eating and sleeping properly, and often take very little exercise. Other causative factors of heart disease can be having too much fatty foods in one's diet, smoking and excessive drinking. All these factors can contribute towards the narrowing and blocking of the arteries and heart attacks.

Heart disease is most common among middle-aged men who are in highly paid professions where there is a lot of stress. Generally it is true to say that men suppress their feelings whereas women express theirs through tears and talking with friends. In contrast to the West where many people die of heart attacks, in the Tibetan community this cause of death is very rare.

TYPES OF HEART DISEASE

There are seven types of heart disease listed in the Tibetan medical texts:

1 *SNying choe* or madness
2 *SNying ser* or angina
3 *SNying tse* or inflammation of the heart
4 *SNying chu* or fluid accumulation in the heart
5 *SNying theb* or depression.

6 *SNying tsin* or heart worm
7 *SNying ne kha le ngakpo* or heart failure

SYMPTOMS OF HEART DISEASE

- Madness
  One becomes forgetful, disorientated, depressed, nervous, short of breath; suffers from sleeplessness, sighing all the time, answering unasked questions, ignoring questions asked and loss of physical co-ordination.
- Angina
  This is divided into two categories. Firstly, if *sNying ser* is caused by the disturbance of *Loong* one will feel dizzy, suffer from pains in the back, experience difficulty in breathing, and there will be dryness on the tongue and in the mouth. Secondly if the *Nying ser* is caused by blood disorder there is severe pain in the chest, breathlessness, fixed staring of the eyes, dry tongue.
- Inflammation of the heart
  One suffers from palpitations, burning sensations in the chest and the back as if there is a flame inside the body, a feeling of one's heart being cut with a knife, dry tongue, dry nose.
- Fluid accumulation in the heart
  One suffers from palpitations, talks excessively, shivering, insomnia, becomes very quick-tempered, laughs continually, listens to songs all the time.
- Depression
  The symptoms are forgetfulness, loss of appetite, worrying for no reason, apathy towards one's life, a feeling inside the body that there is a heavy weight like a large stone, excessive sleep.

- Heart worms
  The colour of the sclera in the eyes becomes black, there are palpitations, uncontrollable dripping of thick saliva, a feeling of being in the dark as if one is living in a cave, a feeling of one's heart being sawed into pieces.
- Heart failure
  One becomes very quiet but irritable, exhibits strange behaviour such as frightening others, suffers from an inability to look out of the sides of the eyes, extreme pain in half of the head and distortion of the mouth.

TREATMENT

Treatment depends on the type of heart disease and in Tibetan medicine we have various herbal formulas to treat patients. Heart problems are an important warning from your body and it means you should slow down and take things easy. You can visualize that half your life has now gone, only half is left so what is the point in pushing yourself all the time? Instead you should do some meditation and yoga, take simple regular exercise such as walking and swimming, as these things can really make a difference. Try to avoid all junk and fatty foods, reduce alcohol consumption and stop smoking.

3) ARTHRITIS

In Tibetan arthritis is called *grum-pu,* meaning the breaking of the joints and bones. The causative factors of arthritic problems are eating too much acidic and oily foods and proteins, which are not properly digested. The essence of nutrients are not then transformed into blood, but turn into a serous fluid instead. This fluid spreads to our joints and affects our muscles, bones, nerves, tendons and ligaments. Another major cause of arthritis is living in a damp and cold climate. As we all know from living in Britain, when the weather becomes damper and colder our joints can become stiffer and ache more. There are six types of arthritis:

1 Arthritis connected with the muscles
2 Arthritis connected with bones
3 Arthritis connected with nerves
4 Arthritis connected with tendons and ligaments
5 Cold arthritis
6 Black arthritis

SYMPTOMS

There are general symptoms of arthritis and as well as the specific symptoms of arthritis related to each of the six different types of arthritis above.

The general symptoms are that in the beginning you will feel as if you are going to get a temperature and there is also a feeling of shivering. Your muscles begin to ache and your skin becomes sensitive, your face becomes oily, there is a feeling of lethargy and it is easy to sweat. All the joints then become stiff and painful. When arthritis becomes very bad there is excruciating pain when moving the body.

The specific symptoms of arthritis connected with the **muscles** are related to *mKhris-pa* and *Bad-Kan* disorders, the joints become very swollen and black in colour, there is numbness in the limbs and it even affects the normal functioning of the heart and lungs. In some extreme cases people will also suffer from nosebleeds and there will be so much pain it will feel as if someone is tearing away the muscles from the bones.

The specific symptoms of arthritis connected with the **bones** are related to *Loong* disorders. There is unbearable pain in the bones, a feeling of thirst, there is difficulty in gaining weight even though the patient has a normal diet. The patient becomes quick-tempered and is unable to bear any loud noise, there is fear of being touched as the bone density of the sufferer is so brittle. From my point of view this form of arthritis is very much connected with the wear and tear of the body and is what is known in Western medicine as osteoarthritis and osteoporosis.

The specific symptoms of arthritis connected with the **nerves** are related to blood disorders. The complexion of the patient becomes very pale and it affects the lungs and heart. The hip-bones are very painful and the surrounding veins of the joints are swollen and painful.

The specific symptoms of arthritis related to the **tendons** and **ligaments** occur when arthritis has become very advanced and as a result the bones and joints have become deformed. There is stiffness and contraction and this has a great effect on normal bodily movements and it can have a devastating effect on day-to-day-life.

The specific symptoms of **cold arthritis** are related to *Loong* and *Bad-Kan*. It is less inflamed and painful and as such it is one of the milder forms of arthritis.

The specific symptoms of **black arthritis** are connected with *mKhris-pa* and blood disorders, both of which are hot in nature. The joints become swollen and painful and according to Western medical science this is what is known as rheumatoid arthritis.

TREATMENT

With regard to diet and lifestyle the arthritis patient should avoid all sour fruits such as lemon, lime, grapefruit, oranges, pineapple, strawberries, gooseberries, blackberries, blackcurrants, plums; vegetables such tomatoes, potatoes and rhubarb; strong cheeses such as Stilton, Danish blue, Cambazola. Salty and fatty foods should also be avoided. All these foods can be like poison to the arthritis sufferer.

With regard to lifestyle it is best to avoid damp conditions and exposure to the cold. If the arthritis is related to *Loong* and *Bad-Kan* disorders, the patient should keep themselves warm, especially the feet and the knees throughout the year, take hot baths, take regular mild exercise such as walking. If the arthritis is connected to blood and *mKhris-pa* disorders the sufferer must avoid too much sun, excessive heat and sleeping in the daytime.

The arthritis patient should eat food such as rice, cereals, pulses, fish, chicken, mango, banana, pears, papaya, ginger, garlic, fresh vegetables, low fat yoghurts and cottage cheese.

I can say with full confidence that Tibetan medicine is one of the best forms of treatment for arthritis. There are various combinations of herbal and mineral medicines such as *acacia 25, Garuda 5, Shorea Robusta 10, Moonseed 5* and *Acacia 23*. Medicines such as *Pomegranate 5* are also prescribed to strengthen the digestive system.

Arthritis is not life threatening but it is a crippling disease which needs perseverance on the part on the patient who chooses Tibetan medicine as a form of treatment. They must be prepared to take the medicine over a long period of time and to take care over diet and lifestyle if their condition is to improve.

4) RESPIRATORY DISEASES

Respiratory diseases are known in Tibetan as *dbugs-mi-bde-ba* which means difficulty in breathing. The causative factor of breathing problems is connected to the digestive system. An excess intake of cold, raw, heavy foods such as milk products, carbohydrates, starchy foods, red meats, exposure of the body to the damp and cold – all of these factors gradually degenerate the digestive heat. This leads to the development of excess undigested particles such as sticky phlegm and mucus which slowly obstruct the respiratory system and cause breathing problems. Other causes are dust pollution, smoking and lack of exercise. There are five types of respiratory disease:

1 *Phran-tshegs* or exertional breathing problems
2 *Mun-can* or bronchitis
3 *Dhugs-chad* or expiratory breathing problems
4 *Chen-po* or gasping
5 *Gen-den* or inspiratory breathing problems

There are general and specific symptoms. The general symptoms for all these types of breathing problems are shortness of breath, pain in the chest and ribs, bloated stomach and, when very severe, the chest becomes relatively silent.

The specific symptoms of **exertional breathing problems** are triggered by just a little physical exertion, over-eating and over consumption of liquids.

The specific symptoms of **bronchitis** are that the bronchial tree is blocked by mucus which leads to the phlegm being constantly expectorated. This strains the throat which in turn affects the voice. The shoulder blades become very stiff and painful and, when lying down, the patient experiences great discomfort.

The specific symptoms of **expiratory breathing problems** are that breathing becomes very difficult, especially exhalation, there is dryness of the mouth and speech becomes broken so that the voice sounds like it is whispering.

The specific symptoms of **gasping** are loss of voice, wheezing, dry throat and there is great effort needed to bring out phlegm, there is a constant feeling of congestion in the chest and a feeling of the need to clear it.

The specific symptoms of **inspiratory breathing problems** are caused by the imbalance of the upward moving *Loong*. *Loong* is unable to move through its own pathways as they are blocked by mucus. It is easier to exhale than it is to inhale and there is a constant lack of air in the lungs, the patient therefore becomes exhausted due to the lungs being starved of air.

TREATMENT

With regard to diet and lifestyle the patient should avoid salty foods such as roasted peanuts, crisps, bacon, deep-fried foods like fish and chips, chillies, processed foods, chilled drinks taken straight from the fridge and ice cream. The patient should try to practise light forms of breathing meditation and relaxation.

When treating patients the physician prescribes medicine to improve digestive absorption and to balance the *Loong* energy in order for the patient to be more relaxed. Medicine is prescribed to strengthen the lungs and bring out the sputum. Medicines can be prescribed in the form of pills and some of the most common ones are *Grape 7*, *Clove 6*, *Gentian 15*, *Buckthorn 19* and *Agar 35*.

5) SKIN DISEASES

The causative factors of skin disease are an unhygienic lifestyle and the intake of excess sugar, citrus, alcohol and illegal drugs. These factors feed the micro-organisms in our body, cause the excess production of impure serums and lead to skin problems. In Tibetan medicine there are nine different types of skin disease:

- Lucoderma
- Eczema
- Warts
- Scabies
- Psoriasis
- Acne

- Freckles
- Patches
- Blemishes

- If lucoderma is connected with *Loong* disorders the skin is a little blackish and dry. If it is connected with *mKhris-pa* disorders the hair falls from the surrounding area on the skin and there is a burning sensation. If it is due to *Bad-Kan* disorders the skin becomes hard and itchy.
- In Tibetan eczema is called *lang-shu* (ox's neck, so named because of the skin condition of the neck of an ox caused by heavy pulling). The skin becomes scaly, inflammed, oozing, there is the thickening of the skin, and vesiculation (small sacs containing liquid form).
- Warts are divided into two – white and black warts.
- Scabies is a contagious skin disorder, the skin colour becomes bluish, there is intense itching and the surrounding hair on the skin falls out.
- Psoriasis is a skin disease where the skin becomes cracked, dry, scaly and itchy. The skin temperature becomes either too cold or too hot.
- Acne is a pimple with a white pus-filled tip.
- Freckles are small brown or black spots on the skin.
- Patches are a skin disease where the patch area becomes whitish and differs from the rest of the skin.
- Blemishes are brown patches which differ from the rest of the skin.

All the above skin diseases are treated according to their own particular types.

6) DIABETES

In Tibetan medicine diabetes is called *gChin-sNyi*, or frequency of urine. It is caused by excessive intake of salt, sugar, cold, heavy and raw foods, also by walking in a cold and damp climate and staying in a damp place for a long period of time. All these factors increase the *Bad-Kan* disorders and strain the kidneys and urinary bladder.

The general symptoms of diabetes are feeling very sleepy, stickiness of the skin all over the body, strong body odour, extreme dryness of the mouth and palate, a craving for cold drinks, burning sensations on the palms and soles of the feet. There is fast growth of hair and nails. The urine is cloudy and thick in density and if urinating outside the urine will immediately attract lots of flies because of the high sugar content. When properly absorbed, sugar helps aid energy and the growth of the tissues. There are three types of diabetes:

The first is *Loong* type diabetes, the symptoms of which are restlessness, palpitations, intense hunger, tiredness, sleeplessness and breathlessness, excess production of phlegm. The urine is oily, sticky and like honey. *Loong* type diabetes is very similar to diabetes mellitus type I in Western terms.

MKhris-pa type diabetes symptoms are infections in the genitalia and urinary bladder, intense thirst, hot bodily temperature, diarrhoea, a constant suffering from influenza. The urine is blackish, bluish, yellowish, red and of strong odour.

Bad-Kan type diabetes symptoms are too much sleep, little appetite, excess production of mucus, vomiting, weight gain. The urine is like sugar cane juice, rice soup, sperm or as clear as water. This type is quite similar to non-insulin dependent diabetes mellitus type II.

If the above diabetes are left untreated and become chronic there will be 10 abscesses which can affect the blood vessels and cause toxins in the blood stream leading to coma, blindness and kidney disorders. Treatment depends on the type of diabetes and there is different advice for diet and conduct for each type.

7) POISONS

According to prophecies in the Tibetan medical texts the age in which we now live is a time when the world's natural resources become very much depleted, and there is great disruption to the environment and the five natural elements. These factors create the causes for 18 new types of malignant diseases which threaten the lives of humans.

COMPOUNDED POISONS

Compounded poisons can be a combination of precious stones such as gold, silver, copper, bronze, iron, lead and mercury and minerals such as iron hydroxide, iron ore, zinc, calcite and sulphur. Such combinations can produce poison which is transmitted through the rays of the sun, smoke, polluted air, physical touch and contaminated food.

FOOD POISONS

Food poisons are caused by wrong combination and incompatible foods, for example, chicken and yogurt and fish and eggs. Also eating something which one is not used to can upset the digestive system and disrupt the seven bodily constituents and three eliminating functions

NATURAL POISONS

Natural poisons can be divided into two: poison from plants and poison from animals.

Poison from plants includes black aconite, yellow aconite, datura, caltrops, spurge and maddar grass. Poison from animals includes snake venom, rabid dog bite, scorpion and bee stings.

If someone accidentally took an aconite overdose the symptoms would be the tongue and limbs becoming numb, burning sensations, the lip and tongue becoming cracked, black complexion, cold breath, fainting, loss of consciousness, stiffness of the limbs and bloated stomach with excruciating pain. The physician would immediately give a herbal combination of natron, tumeric, and myrobalan to stop the poison spreading.

If someone is bitten by a mad dog the dog will look deaf and blind, saliva will be running from its mouth (which will be always open), its head will be bent, its tail inverted and it will wander aimlessly. When someone is bitten by a mad dog the wound turns black/brown and becomes swollen. If it is not treated immediately the patient gets headaches, becomes shivery and delirious, faints, pants, is unable to look in a mirror or in water. When the disease is advanced the human behaves like a dog. For rabies the physician gets toxins out of the system by prescribing medicine such as the *Great Multi-compounded Precious Pill* or the *Great Cold-compounded Precious Black Pill.* Both these precious pills contain more than 70 different types of minerals and herbs as antidotes to the poison. Spiritual help from an advanced tantric practitioner can also be used, they can take the poisons out of the wound by sucking out the poison in the initial stage.

8) CHILDCARE AND CHILDHOOD ILLNESSES

According to the Tibetan medical texts, and in Tibetan society, childcare begins as soon as the child is born. Every parent wants their child to be normal and healthy and for the mother to have an easy labour. The auspicious signs of birth are that the umbilical cord should entwine the upper part of the body, the head should be long and the fontanel should be small. The signs of normal birth are that the head should emerge first, the baby should cry loudly and suck the breast of the mother very energetically. If the legs or buttocks of the baby appear first, if the fontanel is big, and if the baby is unable to suck the mother's breasts, these are signs of abnormal delivery. The signs of inauspicious birth are that the umbilical cord entwines the lower part of the body and that the baby already has teeth.

Once the baby has had a normal birth and is healthy, the parents have to recite the auspicious prayers and words of good luck, such as 'My child, you are like my heart. You are going to live for hundreds of years and you are going to meet great spiritual masters, your life will be full of wealth, good health and fame. I hope there will be no obstacles in your life.' When the recitation is finished the midwife or one of the family members cuts the umbilical cord and ties it with woollen thread; costus powder and sesame oil are then applied to heal the cuts. A special person should then take the baby, hold it in their lap and then wash it with scented lukewarm water. They have to write the sacred Tibetan syllable *HRIH* with saffron powder on the tongue of the baby, this helps generate wisdom and the qualities of good speech.

The baby must be breast fed by the mother with loving kindness so that her milk will easily flow, if she is angry and under stress the milk will not flow properly. If the mother is unable to produce any milk the baby will need to have a wet nurse who should be healthy, kind and who is able to save the life of a baby. In consultation with all the family a good name for the child must be chosen. When the baby is eight months old the ears are pierced, if the baby is a boy it is the right ear which is pierced and if it is a girl it is the left ear. In Tibet earrings are worn by both men and women.

It is important for the baby not to be exposed to strong direct sunlight. Since living in England I have seen many young mothers taking their children out in the sun without adequate protection, this kind of behaviour can sometimes cause eye problems for the child. The fontanel and soles of the feet should also be well protected from the sun as the head is an ocean of nerves and both these areas of the body are connected with sensory nerves inside the head which affect vision. However, if the baby is given an occasional massage in moderate sunlight, this is very good for the baby's growth, circulation and vitality. When lifting the baby it is highly advisable not to lift too early in an upright position, this is because the baby's spine is not strong enough to hold its own head and if forced to do so too soon it will affect the spinal cord and lead to a stooped posture when young.

When the baby is teething it suffers great pain and discomfort throughout the body. The analogy given in the Tibetan medical texts is when a young peacock is growing its head feathers it undergoes great pain and this is similar to the teeth growing inside the baby's mouth. To soothe the baby's discomfort and to relieve the pain in the gums there is a herbal ointment in Tibetan medicine which is based on wild chrysanthemum. If teeth were present at birth a special fire ritual is performed to get rid of any obstacles and bad omens that there might be for the family and child.

Twelve months after the birth there is an anniversary celebration and an offering is made to the three jewels of the Buddha, dharma and sangha. In the past Tibetans have not celebrated any further birthdays in a person's life, however this is now changing due to life in exile and exposure to other cultures. Childhood illnesses are divided into two:

- **Congenital diseases**
- **Common illnesses**

A – CONGENITAL DISEASES

As mentioned in chapter five on human embryology, the mother's diet and conduct during the first three months of pregnancy is crucial for the health and wellbeing of the baby. The mother should not drink alcohol, smoke, take drugs, expose herself to x-rays or exert herself too much through actions such as performing sexual activities frequently or in unusual positions. These can all lead to both disruption of the three principal energies and to blood disorders. These energies are crucial for the development of the foetus and, if disrupted, cause congenital abnormalities such as deafness, blindness, stammering, lameness, spinal deformities and cleft lip. These are all difficult to cure.

B – COMMON ILLNESSES

These can be caused either by improper diet or negligence in care. Illness can result from accidents such as the baby falling from the lap, being bumped or shaken, being forced to stand upright too early, having the umbilical stump pulled off too early, and by excessive crying due to lack of supervision by the parents. Being left on damp ground, not changing nappies on time, giving the baby too much hot potency food such as milk, cream, lamb, garlic or too much cold foods and drinks (such as ice cream). All these factors can be the cause of the 24 different types of childhood illnesses mentioned in the Tibetan medical texts. These different types of illness can be divided into major, minor and very minor illnesses.

Major illnesses can be chest infection, lung and liver diseases, diarrhoea, vomiting, contagious fever, navel infections, urinary stones.

Minor illnesses can be throat infection, spleen and gall bladder illnesses, digestive and colon problems, accumulation of cerebrospinal fluid, geophagia (the habit of eating clay or earth), poisoning through infected milk from the mother's breast.

Very minor illnesses are eye and ear diseases, mouth ulcers, inflammation of the glands, spinal diseases, worms and anal abscesses.

The general symptoms which occur when the baby is not well are constant crying even though the baby has been fed and changed and the crying is not related to teething problems. There will be loss of appetite, tiredness, unwillingness to open the eyes, no interest in playing and breathlessness. If the baby has problems connected with particular organs it will cry very loudly when lifted and touched around that vulnerable part of its body.

DIAGNOSIS

It is difficult to read the baby's pulse, therefore Tibetan physicians have a special way of making diagnoses by reading the ear lobes of the baby. This method of diagnosis is called *na-ta,* or ear map. When being examined by the physician the baby should sit on the mother's lap facing towards the light or the sun. The physician will then stand behind the baby and check the blood vessels of the baby's earlobes. The earlobe is similar in appearance to a leaf from a plant where all its lines are visible. The right earlobe of a baby is divided into three parts; the upper part is diagnosed for the lungs and large intestine, the middle part is for the liver and gall bladder and lower part is for the right kidney and the urinary bladder. The left earlobe is also divided into three parts, the upper part is for the heart and small intestine, the middle part is for the spleen and stomach and the lower part is for the left kidney and reproductive organs.

If any of the above mentioned parts of the earlobes are blackish red it means there is infection or inflammation related to the organ associated with that part of the earlobe. If the lines of the earlobe are pale it means that the illness is related to cold diseases. If the lines of the earlobes cross over each other it means that there is illness due to the influence of spirits. If the lines of the earlobe are regular in pattern and of similar size it indicates that the illness is temporary and not life threatening, and the baby will soon recover. However, if there are no lines at all it means the baby is not going to live long. There is a special medical text called *The Precious Lotus Garland* which goes into this form of diagnosis in great detail. Other methods of general diagnosis for the baby include urinalysis, questioning the mother with regard to signs and symptoms of illness and visual observation.

Once diagnosis has been made the physician will prescribe medicine according to each particular illness and disease. From my experience of seeing children in the West I find that since they are so used to taking Western medicines which are sweetly flavoured, it is very difficult to persuade them to take the bitter tasting forms of Tibetan medicine. However, I do see a number of children who are now used to the strange taste and who take Tibetan medicine very regularly!

9) GYNAECOLOGICAL DISEASES

There are specific, common and obstetric gynaecological diseases.

SPECIFIC GYNAECOLOGICAL DISEASES

Women have a different physical constitution to men. The biggest difference in their bodies is that they have breasts, a uterus and a monthly menstruation cycle and these can bring on a number of gynaecological diseases and illnesses. In the Tibetan medical texts 40 different kinds of specific and common gynaecological disease are mentioned.

The five uterine diseases are related to *Loong, mKhris-pa, Bad-Kan,* blood and a combination of all these together. There are 10 menstrual disorders connected with the lungs, heart, liver, spleen, gall bladder, kidneys, small intestines, heavy period, breasts and absence of any period. There are six chronic menstrual disorders related to bones, heart, kidneys, stomach, small intestine and headaches. These disorders are caused by menstruation and serum concentrated by the *Loong* energy and dispersed into the pathways of nerves and organs.

COMMON AND OBSTETRIC GYNAECOLOGICAL DISEASES

These are morning sickness, abortion, breech birth, obstructions to the ejection of the placenta, prolapse of the uterus, post-natal haemorrhage, post-natal ailments and post-natal infections.

From my experience in the Tibetan community breast cancer and uterine cancer are very rare. This has been attributed to the very little use of modern contraceptive methods for women and due to different lifestyle and diet. For example, the food in India and Tibet is generally organic and contains far less additives and chemicals. Similarly when the women have their periods they have more time to rest as generally they do not have as stressful a lifestyle as women in the West, especially compared to those with careers. Recently I saw a woman who is a lawyer and she told me that she was so busy that she simply did not have time to have her regular period and that she was taking medicines to suppress it. After a long discussion I strongly advised her to at least allow her body to function naturally.

7

METHODS OF DIAGNOSIS

This chapter looks at diagnosis, omens and dreams of impending death, and dealing with disease.

DIAGNOSIS

Just as we can predict that when we see smoke in the distance we know there is a fire, similarly we can predict disease or illness through observing signs and symptoms. However, we need to be cautious when diagnosing illness; when we see a small dark cloud in the sky and predict it is going to rain we might be wrong. Therefore the physician should take time and make their diagnosis only when they are absolutely sure. In Tibetan medicine diagnosis is divided into three sections:

1 Visual observation
2 Touch
3 Questioning

1) VISUAL OBSERVATION

The physician must use all of his or her senses in diagnosis and also closely observe the five senses of the patient in order to diagnose any imbalance of the internal organs. For example, weakness of eyesight means that the liver is weak; if the patient has dry lips and sores it means there is heat in the spleen; if the patient has a hearing problem it might be connected with the kidneys; it there is difficulty in speech it might be connected with the heart; if the patient has nasal problems it might be connected with the lungs. The physician also has to observe the height and weight of the patient and their skin complexion. Also, from my experience, sometimes as soon as a patient enters my consultation room I am able to observe through their body language any stress, anger and unhappiness in their lives. The most important methods of visual observation for the Tibetan physician however, are tongue diagnosis and urinalysis.

TONGUE DIAGNOSIS

The table below lists symptoms of the three *Nyes-pas* that are found through tongue diagnosis.

Table showing disease of the three Nyes-pas and tongue texture

Nyes – pas	Tongue
Loong	Reddish, coarse, dry texture
mKhris-pa	Thick yellowish coating
Bad-kan	Pale, smooth and whitish coating, moist texture

URINALYSIS

This is one of the most unique features of Tibetan medicine in comparison to other forms of ancient medical science. For the Tibetan physician, the urine is like a mirror through which they can observe the internal imbalance and bodily temperature of the patient.

PROCEDURES TO BE FOLLOWED THE NIGHT BEFORE URINALYSIS

The patient has to observe certain preliminary practices before proper urinalysis can be performed by the physician. The night before the urinalysis the patient should avoid strong tea and coffee, alcohol, buttermilk, vitamins and other forms of medication (if possible), spicy foods and food which is heavy and difficult to digest, such as rare steak. The patient should avoid physical exertion such as running, strenuous work such as digging the garden, staying up late and getting little sleep, having too much mental activity, and especially, they should avoid sexual intercourse. All these factors will affect proper diagnosis through urinalysis. If the patient, for example, has eaten hot potency foods such as meat along with spicy foods and has had hot potency drinks such as alcohol, it is possible to mistake their urine with a *mKhris-pa* disorder when they may not have a *mKhris-pa* disorder at all. The patient should therefore drink a moderate quantity of liquid and eat plain vegetarian food such as rice and vegetables, and they should have a good night's sleep with plenty of rest.

The urine sample from which diagnosis is made should be the first early morning urine, any time after midnight. Generally speaking, before midnight all the food and drink from the day is still being digested and eliminated, whilst afterwards, fresh urine will indicate more accurately any kind of internal imbalance and the correct bodily temperature. The urine container should be sterilized and the quantity should be 30 millilitres.

TIME OF URINALYSIS

The best time for the physician to inspect the urine is first thing in the morning under natural light. However this is often impractical for me as I see patients throughout the course of the day and often in the evening (when in winter of course there is no natural light at all). The container in which the urine is analysed should be a white porcelain bowl which is not too deep or shallow and the urine should be stirred by the physician with a thin wooden stick.

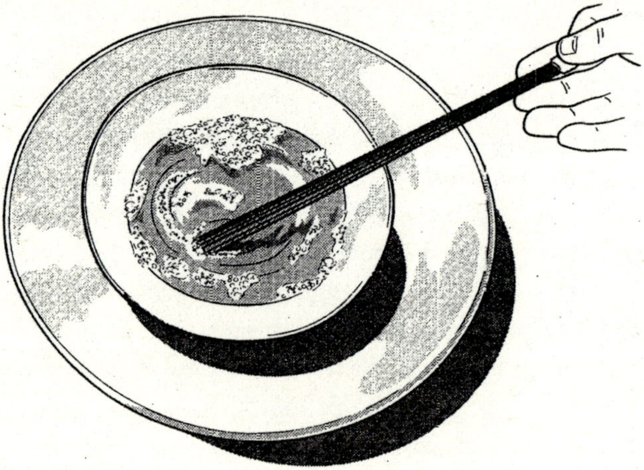

Urinalysis

I have found that urinalysis is always quite difficult to successfully perform. This is due to a number of reasons such as people forgetting to bring a sample, bringing a wrong kind of sample such as one taken in the middle of the afternoon or bringing a sample after not having followed the above procedures.

FORMATION OF URINE

Whatever we eat or drink goes into the stomach where it is absorbed and digested. The waste products go through the small intestine to the large intestine where they are separated into solid and liquid waste products. Liquid goes straight through the kidneys to the urethra and then to the urinary bladder. The essence of food goes to the liver and produces blood, the impurities of blood go to the gall bladder and produces bile. The essence of bile produces serum, and the impurities of bile become the sediments of urine. Because of these factors the intake of food can affect the colour of urine.

HEALTHY PERSON'S URINE

The urine of a healthy person is light yellow in colour, the vapour is neither too strong nor too weak, the urine has bubbles of medium size, the sediment is of average density.

DISEASED PERSON'S URINE

The diseased person's urine has general and specific forms:

General

Generally we check the urine of the diseased person when it is either hot, lukewarm or cold. From my experience so far in the West, all of the urine I have analysed has been cold.

When it is hot, after stirring, we check the colour, vapour, odour and the size of the bubbles. When it is lukewarm, after stirring, we check the sediments and scum (similar to the thin layer which forms on the top of boiled milk). When it is cold, after stirring, we check how long it takes for the bubbles to disperse, the way the bubbles disperse and whether the colour of the urine has changed or not, for example from white to yellow or yellow to white.

Hot urine

For hot urine we look at the colour, vapour, odour and bubbles.

- **Colour** – For the patient with a *Loong* disorder the colour of the urine is bluish, for the *mKhris-pa* patient the urine is yellow and for the *Bad-kan* patient the urine is white. If the urine is red it means there is a blood disorder, if it is light pink it means there is a serum disorder, if the urine is brown it means there is an ulcer, if it is like oil it is because of jaundice, if the urine is black or rainbow-coloured it means it is because of poison. It is also possible for food and drink to affect the colour of the urine, as from my own experience I once saw a patient whose urine was light pink. After reading his pulse I knew there was no serum disorder and upon asking him whether he had had any unusual food he told me that he had eaten beetroot and it was this which had changed the urine colour.

- **Vapour** – If the vapour is profuse it means there is a hot disorder related to *mKhris-pa* and to the blood, if it is small and short-lived it means there is a cold disorder, if it is small and lasting it means there is chronic fever.
- **Odour** – If there is strong odour it means there is a hot disorder, if there is very little odour it is a cold disorder. If there is a smell of a particular food in the urine it means that the food has not been digested properly. In this regard I saw a female patient whose urine smelt strongly of eggs and upon questioning her she told me that she had recently eaten eggs and had felt sick afterwards, and that she had always had a problem digesting eggs. After hearing this I advised her that it would be much easier for her to digest eggs if she made an egg soup with ingredients such as fresh root ginger, coriander seeds, spinach and onions as all these foods aid digestion.
- **Bubbles** – When the urine is stirred if there are big bubbles it means there is a *Loong* disorder, if the bubbles are yellow it is a *mKhris-pa* disorder, if the bubbles are foamy like saliva it is a *Bad-Kan* disorder. If the bubbles are red it is a blood disorder and if the bubbles are rainbow-coloured it is due to poison. If the bubbles scatter immediately when

being stirred, in the same way as a flock of birds scatter in the sky upon the sound of a gunshot, it means that disease has already spread throughout the body.

Lukewarm urine

For lukewarm urine we look at the sediment and scum.

- **Sediment** – When the sediment is thin and long, like hairs, it means there is a *Loong* disorder, if the sediment is like cotton in water it means there is a *mKhris-pa* and blood disorder, if the sediment is short like a hair tip it means there is a *Bad-Kan* disorder. When the sediment is like a cloud it is a lung disorder, if it is very pus-like it means there is pus in the lungs, if the sediment is like sand it means there is a kidney disorder, if it's like golden sand it means there is a urinary obstruction. If a man suffers from premature ejaculation it is possible to detect this in the sediment of his urine; it will be thick and white at the bottom. It is also possible to read the body temperature of the patient by observing the thickness of the urine sediment.
- **Scum** – If the scum is thick it means there is a hot disorder and if it is thin it means there is a cold disorder. If the layer of scum breaks into pieces it means there is a tumour.

Cold urine

- Bubbles – When it is stirred and the bubbles immediately disperse it means there is hot disorder, if the bubbles stay long it means there is cold disorder. If after being stirred the bubbles disperse from the outer rim of the urine bowl it means it is a cold disorder, if the bubbles disperse from the middle of the bowl it is a hot disorder.

- Colour – If the urine becomes more concentrated after being left for a little while it means it is hot disorder and if it remains the same colour it is cold disorder.

Finally when the urine is like blood – its odour like rotten leather or sour milk – it is a sign of impending death. If the urine is blue, has no odour or vapour and the physician observes no changes in the bubbles after checking, the urine is also a sign of impending death.

It is possible to detect and diagnose many different kinds of diseases through performing urinalysis. It is even possible for some experienced Tibetan physicians to diagnose the disease merely by looking at the urine sample and not the patient. In Tibet, due to great distances, it was quite common for urinalysis to be performed in this way when the patient was unable to travel. In today's society where everyone is so busy and our diet and lifestyle so chaotic, it is often very difficult to get a proper urine sample from which diagnosis can be made.

All the above methods of diagnosis are known in Tibetan medicine as knowledge through visual observation.

2) TOUCH

Diagnosis through touch in Tibetan medicine is performed by pulse reading. This is one of the most sophisticated methods of diagnosis in Tibetan medicine. It takes years to learn and decades to fully master. The pulse is like a messenger between the physician and the disease. The preliminaries to be observed on the part of the patient for a proper pulse reading are the same as those for urinalysis. In the Tibetan medical texts pulse reading is divided into thirteen sections. Here I will just give a general overview.

TIME OF PULSE READING

The proper time to read the pulse is first thing in the morning. The patient should not move from their bed and their stomach should be empty. In the human body there are three main subtle channels known in Tibetan as *rkyang-ma, roma* and *Bu-ma*. The *rkyang-ma* channel is influenced by the moon, *roma* by the sun and *Bu-ma* by neutral energy. At night the pulse beat is slower because the lunar influence is stronger, and in the daytime the pulse is faster and stronger because the solar influence is stronger. At dawn, however, when the lines on the palms are visible, these influences are in a dynamic state of equilibrium and therefore this is the best time to read the pulse.

These days of course it is very impractical to read the pulse at such an early time in the morning; however pulse reading can be accurately performed at any time during the course of the day. When I see patients I always tell them to relax for at least 10 minutes before I read their pulse. This is because people often arrive to see me for a consultation after having travelled for many miles and suffered from the stresses caused by the unpredictability of our modern forms of transport, and simply from life in general. It is also very important for the physician to be as relaxed as possible at the time of performing pulse reading.

LOCATION OF PULSE READING

The pulse can be read from any part of the body, such as the jugular pulse in the neck, the abdominal pulse in the abdomen, the dorsal pulse on the ankle, or the heart pulse on the heart. However, if a pulse – such as the heart pulse – is read at a location too close to the heart organ it will be like trying to hold a conversation with people while sitting next to a television which is on at full volume. The physician will simply be unable to understand what the conversation is about. Similarly if the pulse is read at a location which is too far from the organs of the body, such as reading the dorsal pulse on the ankle, it will be like watching the television when the volume is too low to understand anything.

Therefore the most accurate location of pulse reading is on the radial artery on the first crease of the wrist; this location is neither too far from the major bodily organs or too near. This is like sitting comfortably on your sofa and watching your favourite movie with the volume just right. The radial artery is like a newsroom from where reporters have been despatched to many different parts of the country to gather all kinds of news, and they will sometimes bring good news, funny news, serious news and bad news. In a similar way the radial artery is connected with the five vital organs and six hollow organs in our body, and it is read in order to see what imbalance there is in these organs. Two other pulses are also read by the Tibetan physician. These are the ulna artery to read the life span of the patient and the dorsal artery to confirm death.

PRESSURE PLACED ON THE PULSE BY THE PHYSICIAN

As the radial artery lies deep within the wrist, the Tibetan physician will use the six fingers of the index, middle and rings of hands of both hands to read it. The index finger is pressed lightly to feel the skin, the middle finger is pressed with medium pressure to feel the muscle tissue and the ring finger is pressed hard to feel the bone.

HOW TO READ THE PULSE

For pulse reading the fingers of the physician should be supple and at the right temperature. If the patient is male the physician's right hand reads the left arm of the patient. The index finger reads the heart and small intestine (fire element), the middle finger reads the spleen and stomach (earth element) and the ring finger reads the left kidney and reproductive organs

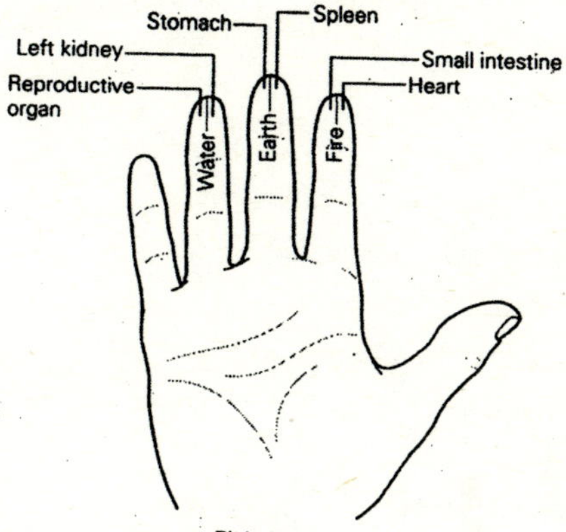

Right hand

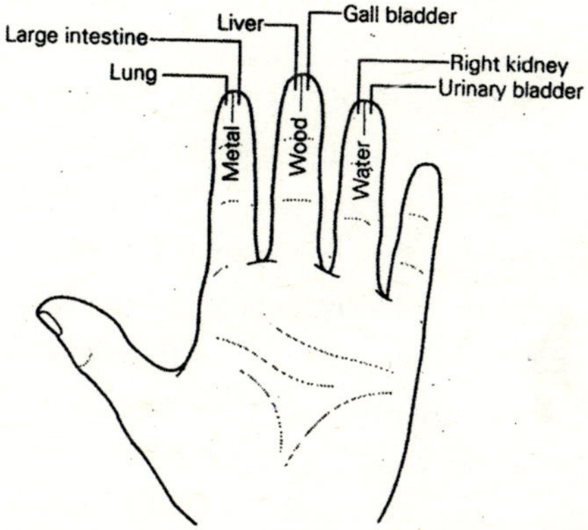

Left hand

Exhibiting the Physician's fingertips with regard to pulse reading

(water element). The physician's left hand then reads the right arm of the male patient. The index finger reads the lung and large intestine (metal element), the middle finger reads the liver and gall bladder (wood element) and the ring finger reads the right kidney and urinary bladder (water element). If the patient is female the right arm is read first and the left arm afterwards.

DIFFERENT PULSES

1 Constitutional pulse
2 Seasonal pulse
3 Substitutional pulse
4 Healthy and diseased pulse
5 General and specific pulse
6 Death pulse
7 Pulse of demonic possession[1]
8 Lifespan pulse

1) Constitutional pulse

The constitutional pulse is the natural beat of your pulse according to your own body constitution when you are healthy and your body is in equilibrium. The three constitutional pulses are male, female and neutral. This does not mean that males have the male pulse and females have the female pulse, it is possible for each to have either. The male pulse is thick and bulky, the female pulse is thin and fast and the neutral pulse is smooth and supple. It is important for the physician to identify the constitutional pulse, otherwise it will be mistaken for the male as *Loong*, the female as *mKhris-pa* and neutral as *Bad-Kan*.

In the medical texts it says that when the physician reads the pulse, if a male happens to have a female pulse it means his life span is long, if the female has a male pulse it means she will have many sons. If a couple both have a neutral pulse it means they will enjoy a long life together and good health, but they will have problems with their close relatives and they will have no offspring. If both partners have a male pulse they will have many sons but no daughters, if both have a female pulse they will have many daughters but no sons. If one partner has a male or female pulse and the other a neutral pulse it means they will have just one child.

2) Seasonal pulse

The Tibetan astrological calendar has 360 days divided into four seasons: spring, summer, autumn and winter. Each season has three months and each month 30 days.

In pulse reading the first 72 days of the spring season (which in the Tibetan calendar is the first three months of the year) have a strong influence on the liver pulse and gall bladder pulse, with wood predominating the season. This is followed by 18 days with the earth element having special influence on the stomach and spleen pulse. Similarly the first 72 days of summer have a strong influence on the heart pulse and small intestine pulse, with the fire element predominating the season. The first 72 days of autumn have a strong influence on the lung pulse and large intestine pulse, with the metal element predominant. Finally, the first 72 days of winter have a strong influence on the pulses of the kidneys, urinary bladder and reproductive organs, with the water element predominant. For each of these last three seasons the earth element also predominates for the last 18 days.

It is important for the physician to know the exact season when checking the pulse otherwise in the summer, for example, the physician may confuse the stronger pulse of the heart and small intestine with disease. Because of this in the medical texts it is said the physician must identify the correct season through observation of external changes such as the position of the stars, the different birds and the appearance of trees.

3) Substitutional pulse

The substitutional pulses are read when the patient is not within reach of the physician, and the physician reads the pulse of a close family member instead. This was performed in Tibet because there were no modern means of communication and a close family member of the patient was then used as a substitute for diagnosis to be made if the patient was unable to see the physician themselves.

4) Healthy and diseased pulse

When the physician reads the pulse its frequency will determine whether the patient is healthy or not. The frequency of the pulse is measured by the inhalation and exhalation of the physician. For healthy people, when the physician inhales the pulse beat should be two and likewise when the physician exhales. In-between inhalation and exhalation the pulse beat should be one, making five in total. This pulse beat should be measured for a long time. If the pulse is more than five the person has a hot disease and if the pulse beat reaches 10 in one inhalation and exhalation of the physician it means the patient has a very high fever, if it reaches seven the patient has a medium fever. If the pulse beat is less than five the person has a cold disease, and if the pulse drops to only two it means the patient is extremely weak and has a very serious cold disease.

5) General and specific pulse

General pulse is divided into cold and hot. The characteristics of hot pulse are divided into six: strong pulse, overflowing pulse, rolling pulse, fast pulse, twisted pulse, firm pulse. The characteristics of cold pulse are also divided into six: weak pulse, sunken pulse, declining pulse, slow pulse, loose pulse, empty pulse.

For specific pulse with regard to the three principal energies, if it is a *Loong* disorder the pulse is floating, empty and halting; if it is a *mKhris-pa* disorder the pulse is thin and twisted; and if it is a *Bad-Kan* disorder the pulse is slow and sunken.

With regard to other diseases, if a patient has a blood disorder the pulse is bumpy and rolling, if they have a lymph disorder the pulse is shaky and moves with difficulty, if it is a leprosy pulse it will be trembling and thrilling, if the pulse is due to compounded poisons it is rough, short and difficult to feel, and if it is due to meat poison it is thin, fast, sunken and missing.

6) Death pulse

For death the pulse is halting, irregular, missing and changeable. If the heart pulse is missing the patient will live for one day, if the lung pulse is missing they will live for only two days, if the liver pulse is missing they will live for three days, if the spleen pulse is missing they will live for five days and if the kidney pulse is missing they will live for eight days.

7) Pulse of demonic possession

Signs indicative of demonic possession are a sudden and erratic pulse, or concurrent, halting and pulling pulses. When the physician feels this form of pulse they will immediately recommend that the patient sees a spiritual practitioner who will be able to perform the appropriate rituals to banish the evil spirit.

8) Life span pulse

The life span pulse is read at the ulna artery. The ulna pulse should beat regularly and not be too strong or too weak. If the pulse beats continuously one hundred times it means the person will live for 100 years, if it beats continuously fifty times the person will live for 50 years.

Pulse reading is the most complicated and subtle method of diagnosis in Tibetan medicine and in Tibetan medicine it is known as *che pa thun gyi rigpa* or intuitive knowledge of diagnosis.

3) QUESTIONING

The physician needs to have a sympathetic ear and realize the fact that the patient will have come to visit them full of hope that they might be cured, while at the same time full of anguish because of their illness. It is best if the physician is a good listener and open-minded, but also mindful that the relationship between a physician and patient is a confidential one. The patient must feel comfortable and relaxed in order for there to be good communication between the patient and the physician. Trust and understanding between the physician and patient is crucial if the patient is to be helped.

From my own experience this method of diagnosis is the most informative. When I see a patient I ask about their medical history, how their illness began, the location of the illness and signs and symptoms of the illness.

The dialogue below is an example of the method of questioning I use when I see new patients. In this particular case the patient is a young man in his mid-twenties.

Question (Doctor) : Please give me a brief medical history.

Answer (Patient) : I had all the usual childhood illnesses, but since having glandular fever about six months ago I have been suffering from fits.

Q : Have you consulted your GP over this?

A : No

Q : Is there any particular time when you have these fits?

A: It always happens at night

Q : So how is your sleep?

A : Terrible. At the most I get two or three hours.

Q : Do you think a lot at night?

A : Yes, that is the only quiet time I have to think.

Q : What is your job?

A : I'm a part-time music student and part-time residential social worker looking after mentally ill people.

Q : Do you drink alcohol?

A : Not now, because when I drink my fits become more frequent.

Q : What is your weight?

A : I don't know but I am always underweight.
Q : Do you feel tired a lot of the time?
A : Always.
Q : How is your concentration?
A : Poor.
Q : Are you doing any exercise?
A : Lots of cycling.
Q : Have you consulted any other alternative practitioner?
A : I have been seeing an acupuncturist and I have taken Chinese medicine. (Shows a decoction.)
Q : What was their diagnosis?
A : That I have heat in my liver.
Q : What is your diet?
A : I'm afraid I have a bad diet.

Following this I read his pulse and performed urinalysis. The pulse was floating, empty when pressed (like an inflated balloon), his liver pulse was very fast and strong, his stomach pulse was very slow and sunken. His urine was pale yellow with big bubbles which disappeared quickly.

My diagnosis was that his problem was due to an imbalance of *Loong* and this was related to his care work job where he often had to deal with people who were in distress and frequently crying and screaming. The glandular fever had affected his liver and spleen which in turn affected his blood circulation and digestive system. Because the man was in his twenties his body was reaching its peak energy where it is dominated by *mKhris-pa* which is hot in nature. The general function of *Loong* is to carry the blood and nutrients throughout the body and when this subtle flow of *Loong* becomes disrupted (in this case because of mental stress and slow circulation) it constricts the blood vessels and nerves in the brain. This was the cause of the young man's fits.

I prescribed a month course of Tibetan herbal medicine for him, to help balance his *Loong* energy and strengthen his liver and digestive system, and also to help improve his sleep pattern.

When I gave him advice on diet he was surprised when I told him to stop eating garlic as he had been eating a lot of garlic because he was under the impression that it would help his condition. I told him that people often only know the positive aspects of garlic and not the negative. Garlic is a very hot potency food and since the young man's bodily nature was already hot, his eating garlic was like putting more logs on the fire, this also applied to alcohol and the fact that when he drank his fits got worse. My other dietary advice was to tell him to avoid hot potency foods such as lamb, nuts and chillies, and fatty foods such as full cream milk and full fat cheese and cream. I told him that he should also avoid light and cool potency foods such as tea and coffee, and that if he did take them it should be before lunch. The foods and drinks which I advised him to take were fresh fruit and fruit juice, herbal teas, lots of vegetables and pulses, rice and other cereals, fish and chicken. Spices such as fresh root ginger and coriander seed could be added to his food to aid his digestion.

With regard to conduct I told him not to force himself to do too much as he had a tendency to want to please everyone at the neglect of himself. I advised him to do some breathing meditation and walking exercise as opposed to cycling which was too strenuous at that time of year (it was the peak of the summer).

OMENS AND DREAMS OF IMPENDING DEATH

Within the Tibetan Buddhist cycle of life there is birth, ageing and disease, and death.Tibetan medical science is able to detect impending death through various signs of physical decay, and these signs are divided into four categories:

1 Long-term signs of decay
2 Short-term signs of decay
3 Uncertain signs
4 Certain signs

1) LONG-TERM SIGNS OF DECAY

Long-term signs of decay can be observed through dreams, thoughts and actions, and physical appearance, and also through messengers (in Tibet if a patient was too ill to see a doctor in person, they would send a messenger).

DREAMS

In Tibetan medicine dreams are characterized into six types:

- Seeing dreams – this type of dream occurs when you have seen something in the daytime and then you dream about it that night.
- Hearing dreams – this type of dream occurs when you have heard something in the daytime or just before going to bed. The dream is then influenced by that sound.
- Feeling dreams – when asleep you feel a soft, hard, light or heavy material and the physical sensation associated with this can influence the content of your dream.
- Praying dreams – this type of dream occurs when you strongly wish or pray for something to happen and then you dream about it.
- Dream of disease – when you are unwell and sick you then also dream about sickness and illness.
- Negative and positive dreams.

Negative dreams occur when the channel of consciousness is blocked by the disruption of the three *nyes-pas*. Because of this the functioning of mind and body becomes disturbed and this leads to negative dreams. Negative dreams can include: riding on a cat, monkey, tiger, jackal, corpse, buffalo, pig, donkey or camel whilst naked and proceeding in a southerly direction. Also negative are dreams of having a bird's nest on top of your head, a tree growing from your head, a thorny tree growing from your heart, a lotus flower blooming out from your heart, falling from a precipice, sleeping in a cemetery, skin peeling and falling away from the limbs, entering the womb, drowning in mud and being carried away by a flood, being swallowed by a fish, finding precious stones, getting married, sitting naked while shaving or cutting your hair, partying with deceased relatives, wearing red clothes, being dragged by dogs. If these are dreamt continuously around the time of dawn then they can be interpreted as being long-terms signs of physical decay.

Positive dreams can include wearing clean white clothes, carrying ceremonial banners, the enthronement of a king or queen, meeting your spiritual masters, witnessing a big fire burning, seeing a clear blue ocean, finding apricots or walnuts, climbing high mountains or onto the roof of a house, climbing a tree abundant with fruit, riding a lion, elephant, horse, or riding cattle, swimming across rivers, travelling in a north easterly direction, escaping from prison or from dark caves, dreaming of gods and goddesses, being praised by one's parents, or performing a religious ceremony. If these are dreamt constantly and at dawn they can be interpreted as being indicative of good health, long life and material gain. These dreams are a warning sign if they are dreamt constantly around the time of dawn, otherwise the above five do not necessarily mean anything.

THOUGHTS AND ACTIONS

If a person's thoughts and behaviour change dramatically – from being calm to being violent or from being violent to calm, from being shy to talkative or from moody to happy – it is a sign of long-term physical decay. In our community in South India we had a neighbour who was in the Tibetan army and who was in his mid-forties. Normally he was very serious and unapproachable, however, one year there was a village party and he surprised everyone by dancing continuously and singing all night. I remember that at the time my mother remarked that this was not normal and that it was not a good sign. She was right as shortly afterwards the man died suddenly.

Similarly if a person suddenly begins to criticize their physician, spiritual teacher, friends and family, and if as a patient they refuse to take any medicine, these are signs of decay; as is quickly gaining a lot of wealth. With regard to these signs I had a patient who was a devoted Buddhist for many years and who I had treated for quite some time. Suddenly he completely changed his attitude towards his teacher and began to heavily criticize him, he also complained about the medicines he was taking from many different physicians. He told me his dreams and that he had nightmares, and he also told me that he felt certain he was going to die. Although he was only a young man he did in fact die very shortly after this.

APPEARANCE

Signs to do with appearance can be when after bathing the region of skin around the heart is dry while the rest of the skin is still wet, the soundless cracking of knuckles when usually there is a sound, the non-appearance of a body shadow in the sun, a headless reflection in the mirror or water, a reflection with limbs missing and the distorted appearance of sense organs such as mouth and ears. As when you see a flower on a fruit tree you know that the fruit will grow, or when you see a dark cloud you know it will rain, it is the same with these appearance changes in that they are the long-term warning signs of decay.

In Tibet when it was not possible for the practitioner to see the patient (due to distance or severity of illness), the practitioner would read the messenger for signs. Consequently the messenger would often be a friend or a family member. If the messenger was in a panic when they reach the physician, looked nervous, or arrived on a date which is astrologically inauspicious, these were seen as signs of decay for the patient.

2) SHORT-TERM SIGNS OF DECAY

Short-term signs of decay can be observed in connection with the five elements and their dissolution in the human body.

- Earth is absorbed by water and vision becomes blurred
- Water is absorbed by fire and causes the bodily cavities to dry up
- Fire is absorbed by air and there is loss of bodily heat
- Air is absorbed by space and respiration ceases

Short-term signs of decay are also observed in the diminishing of the powers of the five sensory organs, this is seen by observing various external physical signs.

- The sense of sight diminishes – vision becomes blurred, and the eyes roll upwards.
- Hearing diminishes – the patient is unable to hear anything and the ears become cupped.
- Smell diminishes – the patient is unable to smell anything and the nostrils become distended.
- Taste diminishes – the patient is unable to taste anything

and there is loss of speech, the tongue becomes dry and black in the middle, the lower lip hangs down and the upper lip rolls upward.

- The sense of touch diminishes – the patient is unable to feel anything.

From the Tibetan Buddhist perspective this is now a crucial moment for deciding the patient's future rebirth, therefore it is very important that the patient has a calm mind. In Tibetan communities spiritual practices such as reciting and reading from Buddhist scriptures like the *Bardo Thodol* would be performed in order for the patient to die as peacefully as possible.

3) UNCERTAIN SIGNS

Uncertain signs of death occur when inauspicious dreams arise during illness. However when the illness ceases so do the dreams.

4) CERTAIN SIGNS

Certain signs of death are internally when the patient is unable to take food and externally when there is only bone and no muscle, no pulse beat and no response to any form of treatment.

In Tibetan society it is vital for a qualified physician to be able to detect and correctly predict impending death in order for the family of the deceased to make the necessary religious preparations.

Tibetans believe in rebirth and the period of 49 days after death is important for the deceased with regard to their next life. However, rebirth of the deceased really depends on their actions in the life which has just ended. For Tibetans the death of a person is not the end and there is much still to be done to help them. It is looked upon as a good time for grieving for the family and friends; they make every effort to perform various religious rites and ceremonies on behalf of the deceased in order to help them. Evidence that this can help is illustrated in the life of Tibet's great yogi Milarepa. Once he was meditating in a cave and that year there was a heavy snowfall for many weeks which blocked the path leading up to it. The local villagers thought he had died and therefore performed the necessary religious ceremonies for the deceased. However, after some time Milarepa appeared, much to the astonishment of the villagers, who told him they thought he had died and that they had performed the usual rituals for him as a deceased. He commented that exactly because they had performed these rituals he had not felt hungry and was able to survive without food.

During this 49 day period the family will try not to show too much emotion as Tibetans believe that the spirit of the dead person will still be inhabiting the places of their previous life. This means that when serving tea the cup of the deceased will also be filled (in Tibetan society each person has their own cup), in order not to upset the spirit.

Immediately after death every effort is made by the family to contact a highly realized lama who can perform *phowa*. This is a method of ejecting the consciousness of the deceased from the body and directing it towards a better rebirth. It can only be successfully performed by a very highly realized practitioner.

Astrologers also play an important role during this period. When someone dies an astrologer is consulted in order to calculate the right day for cremation and which Tibetan Buddhist deities are to be supplicated. The astrologer also checks to see if the deceased is still strongly attached to any family members or possessions. With regard to this I have an example from my own community in South India. One of our neighbours died at what was calculated to be a very inauspicious time. Soon after this the young daughter of the man who died said that on a number of occasions she had seen her father. She was then attacked by one of their cows, of which she still bears the scars to this day. It was during this time that my mother had a dream of a new pair of trousers which were in the house of the deceased and which were moving as if someone was inside them. Normally when someone dies, their clothes and possessions are offered to the local monasteries, and in regard to this my mother asked the wife of the man whether she had kept any of his clothes, especially any trousers. The woman was shocked to hear this from my mother as she had left a new pair of trousers which had belonged to her dead husband and which she had intended to give to his brother. The trousers were immediately offered to the local monastery and after this the disturbances ceased.

One year after the death of the person there is an anniversary known in Tibetan as *Lo Cho* when final farewells are said to the deceased, and again religious rites and rituals are performed. Because of their cultural and religious beliefs, Tibetans are quite accepting of death. When I was growing up in my village my father's generation would carry the dead bodies of the villagers who died to the cemetery where they were cremated. Now when I go back to see my family it is my brothers' generation, who were born and brought up in India, who now do this after having been taught by the older generation. It means they see death at an early age and they have no fear of it. There is a Tibetan proverb which says 'There is no escape if your time is up, even if you are the only son of an enlightened physician'.

DEALING WITH DISEASE

There are nine methods and metaphors for dealing with disease:

1 When the physician needs to confirm diagnosis they can, for example, confirm a *mKhris-pa* disorder by giving a decoction of felwort. If the patient responds positively then there is a *mKhris-pa* disorder. Throughout this process of confirmation the physician should be as cautious as a cat.

2 Once the physician has confidence in their diagnosis they can explain the causes, symptoms and treatment of the disease to the patient, as if they were hoisting a banner on the top of a mountain.

3 Some diseases such as hidden fever require the physician to prescribe a hot potency medicine to bring the fever out. The fever can then be treated with cool potency medication to fully eradicate it. This can be compared to taming a wild horse and putting it in a stable.

4 If the patient comes to the physician after having previously seen another doctor the physician will have to ascertain whether the previous doctor prescribed medication which was either too strong or too mild, or prescribed the wrong medication. For this the physician has to investigate the disease like a gull-catching fish.

5 If the disease is very serious, such as fully developed fever, the physician has to act immediately and treat it with the four water therapies which are dietary instructions such as fasting by taking only water and no solid food, cooling conduct by taking cold baths, medicine given such as camphor decoction and surgery (such as blood-letting from the external jugular vein). This is compared to meeting your enemy in a narrow lane where there is no retreat or escape.

6 Minor diseases are treated gradually by advising on diet, behaviour, prescribing medicine and performing surgery.

This can be compared to a set of stairs that are slowly climbed one after the other.

7 Individual diseases such as *Loong* disorders can be treated separately without disturbing either *mKhris-pa* or *Bad-Kan*. This can be compared to a warrior destroying an enemy on the spot.

8 Multiple or combined diseases such as combinations of *Loong*, *mKhris-pa* and *Bad-Kan* should be treated with equanimity. This can be compared to a cheftain making peace between two disputing parties.

9 It is very important for the physician to consider the patient's bodily constitution, just as it is foolish to put the load of a *dzo* (crossbreed of bull and female yak) on the back of a sheep.

8

TREATMENT TECHNIQUES – PART I

The next two chapters will look at treatment in Tibetan medicine. This first part gives an overall view on diet and conduct.

When taking treatment the patient often assumes that it is solely the responsibility of the physician to cure them, but this is not the case. When seeing patients I always stress to them that it is a team effort. It is like a football team: to have success you need a good manager, good discipline, good diet and good players. The manager has to give proper instruction and guidance to the players but they also have to listen and take responsibility if they are to win. So in this way patients have to listen to the advice of the physician on changing their diet, lifestyle and regularly taking the medicine at the right times. Only after this will there be a positive result. I tell my patients that Tibetan medicine is not a 'quick fix' form of treatment and that it requires patience and perseverance on their part for it to succeed.

Peter, who is one of my patients and is in his early seventies, came to see me with regard to a number of physical complaints. He was suffering from excess perspiration, haemorrhoids, digestive problems and he also needed to improve the grip of his right hand. This was poor due to his right little finger being operated on because of Dupuytren's contraction. The condition was also present in the left little finger which was bending over with a small lump at the base. Because of this illness his other fingers had been damaged and he was unable to write. Due to the fact that he had been in the army where life is very disciplined, he found it difficult to relax mentally and to just not do anything. All of these problems caused him a lot of anxiety.

However, for a number of years now he has been regularly taking Tibetan medicine and closely following my advice with regard to his diet and lifestyle. In fact since he begun his treatment he has never missed a single dose of his medicine! Peter's perseverance and commitment to the treatment has allowed his overall condition to improve. His grip, for example, has improved tremendously and he is now able to write with no problems, the lump at the base of his left finger has disappeared, his haemorrhoids have stopped bleeding, and he is now able to enjoy the changes of the seasons (previously he perspired too much in the summer and winter because of excess bodily heat). As his physical condition has improved so has his mental attitude and he now enjoys an excellent quality of life for a man in his seventies, and he looks many years younger. I really admire his dedication and perseverance. It is important to realize that illnesses develop in our bodies very slowly and over many years and therefore they cannot be immediately cured in a short period of time.

ADVICE ON DIET

In the Tibetan medical texts it says that no matter how much you pull on the bow, the target remains the same size as the tip of the arrow. Similarly farmers work hard throughout the four seasons to cultivate their land but their basic needs are simply to have good food and adequate clothing. We in the West work for eight hours each day, often having to commute in and out of big cities, catch trains and buses and have to put up with all the stresses which these entail. If at the end of all this we eat the wrong foods it is very sad.

Over the last forty years the Western diet has changed quite dramatically for the worse. This is because of modern methods of food production which include the use of growth hormones in animals, preservatives, artificial colourings and flavourings, high usage of fat, salt and sugar contents in products, food processing, and the use of antibiotics to boost nutrition. For example, it is totally unethical to feed a vegetarian animal with processed offal and this can be seen as one of the reasons why we have had so many problems with mad cow disease in England. So all of these factors can deplete food quality.

When I first arrived in this country from India I was very impressed with the cleanliness, choice and presentation of the food available to buy. Once, when I was invited to dinner, the dessert was strawberries and cream. I was amazed at the size of the strawberries as in Dharamsala, where I studied Tibetan medicine, we used to go and pick strawberries and they were tiny, but very sweet and tasty. I was therefore very disappointed at the taste of these large strawberries which in comparison to the ones in India, were watery and tasteless. This was a shock to me and from then onwards I became much more observant of what is contained in the foods for sale in this country. We might have quantity and the ability to make everything look attractive but the quality of the food is often poor.

We are overfed but undernourished. Each of us has a responsibility to promote the use of real organic foods which I notice are now becoming more available. If we continue to demand it, more organic food will be produced and as a result our next generation will be healthier.

In the *rGyud-bzhi* there is great emphasis on dietary principles, and there are three whole chapters devoted to diet. They deal with classification of foods and drinks, their use, precautionary advice, and instruction on consuming the right quantity of food and drink. In Tibet there was not a great choice of fruit and vegetables and therefore in this section I have added things which are not mentioned in the Tibetan medical texts but which are relevant to us now. Diet can divided into food and drink.

FOOD

Food is divided into five categories:

1 Grains
2 Meats
3 Oils
4 Vegetables, fruits and spices
5 Cooked foods

1) GRAINS

Grain is divided into cereals and pulses.

Cereals

- Barley – this is the staple food of Tibet where the barley is roasted and milled to produce *tsampa*. Once the barley is roasted it is very easy to digest and very nutritious. It is high in fibre and helps to clear the bowels.
- Wheat – high in protein and it helps to balance *Loong* and *mKhris-pa*. I have noticed that in this country many people have wheat allergies and I think that if the wheat was milled and roasted properly, it would be much easier to digest.
- Oats – high in calcium, potassium and magnesium, oats are very nutritious and easy to digest. A bowl of hot porridge

in the cold winter is the best breakfast for your mind and body.

- Millet – high in protein, easy to digest and good for *Loong*. It is gluten free and therefore can be used as a replacement for wheat.
- Rice – the easiest cereal to digest, gluten free and rich in protein and vitamin B. It stops diarrhoea and vomiting and it increases virility. However eating too much white rice can cause constipation.
- Buckwheat – strengthens the blood vessels and varicose veins, helps blood pressure, but inflames wounds.

All cereals are sweet in taste and their post-digestive taste is also sweet. Generally they help to strengthen our body and nourish our mind and they help reduce *Loong* disorders.

Pulses

Pulses are an excellent source of soluble fibre and they are a great replacement for protein for the vegetarian. I have great respect for vegetarianism and if vegetarians balance their diet with milk products, cereals and pulses they will be perfectly healthy and there is less risk of suffering cancer and heart disease. From a Buddhist point of view it is also said that if you refrain from killing other beings you will live longer.

- Peas – green beans and peas are easy to digest and help relieve constipation. They need to be steamed and cooked and not taken raw as they can cause flatulence due to a chemical called lectin.
- Moong beans – these are beneficial for male sexual potency, they reduce *Loong* and they contain folic acid which is good for pregnant women.

- Black-eyed beans – they are high in fibre and they contain selenium. They reduce mucus production, help the relief of asthma, piles and urinary stones.
- Soya beans – they are an excellent source of protein, they are low in fat and good for the heart and for blood cholesterol, they are also a cancer preventing food. There are many foods produced from soya beans such as tofu, soya yoghurt and soya milk (which is a great replacement for cows' milk).
- Kidney beans – they are high in fibre, potassium and zinc. When preparing them they must be soaked for a minimum of eight hours and they should then be cooked slowly until they are tender. Otherwise they will cause stomach upsets because they contain lectin which is a toxin.
- Lentils – lentils are the easiest pulse to digest and they are also the most delicious; for example a wonderful dal soup can be made from them. In India, lentils are the major source of protein for vegetarians. They help diabetes, cholesterol and they contain vitamin B. Gout sufferers should avoid lentils as they contain a compound called purine which can create uric acid. However if lentil paste is applied to the infected joints such as the big toes and elbows it will help to reduce the pain. Lentil paste also helps to relieve sufferers of a skin condition called erysipelas.

All pulses should be well cooked and I strongly advise that the following ingredients should be added to them when they are being prepared for eating. These ingredients are fresh root ginger, coriander, coriander seeds, cumin, fennel, garlic – all these will aid the digestion of the pulses and break down their proteins. It is always better to buy pulses dry and not in tins.

2) MEATS

Meat is a great source of first class protein but we must realize that we do not need to eat every kind of meat in order to have a healthy diet. We can live quite easily with a minimum of meat consumption. Different meats have different potencies and we therefore have to be aware of the right kind of meat to eat according to the season.

- Lamb – this meat has the warmest potency and it is very nutritious. It is good for anaemia, it pacifies *Loong* and it increases appetite and energy. It is an excellent meat to eat in the winter but not so much in the hot summer.
- Beef – this meat has a very balanced potency. It is nutritious, helps anaemia and fevers related to *Loong* disorders. Beef can be eaten at any time of the year.
- Pork – has a very cooling potency. It helps to relieve ulcers but it is not good for insomnia and the kidneys. It is good to eat pork in the summer; however if you have high blood pressure and any lung disorders it is best to avoid bacon.
- Goat meat – this also has a very cooling potency. It helps the healing of burns and wounds but it is not good for insomnia. Goat meat can be eaten in the summer.
- Buffalo – it has a warm potency. Buffalo meat increases sleep and weight. When I worked at the Tibetan Medical Institute's clinic in Delhi the only meat available was buffalo and I remember always sleeping like a log.
- Yak – the yak is native to Tibet and it has many benefits for the Tibetans. It only survives and flourishes in lands of high altitude and it is an excellent beast of burden. It is able to walk through snow without any problem due to its thick fur and really a yak is more or less like a buffalo with fur. Yaks can be used by farmers when ploughing their fields and their long thick fur can be used to make slings, tent

ropes, waterproof blankets, rugs, bags, and weather-proof tents for nomads. There is a common misconception in the West that there are such things as yak's milk and butter, however a yak is a male animal and therefore of course it does not produce these!

- Yak meat has warm potency and is most nutritious. It helps the digestive system and kidneys; however if eaten in excess it disrupts *mKhris-pa* and causes blood disorders.
- Chicken – chicken has warm potency and it helps virility and the healing of wounds. Chicken is best eaten in the winter.
- Rabbit – rabbit meat has a very rough potency and helps increase bodily heat and stops diarrhoea.
- Fish – fish has a balanced potency and is excellent for improving digestive heat, eyesight, memory, shrinking tumours, healing wounds and increasing appetite.
- Crab – crab meat has warm potency and it strengthens the kidneys and eliminates water retention.
- Organs - goat's liver is an excellent eye tonic and other animal organs such the lungs, liver, kidney and heart are good to strengthen related human organs; for example if you have weak kidneys you can eat lamb's kidneys.

Generally the upper part of animal meat is much easier to digest than the lower part. For example, lamb's shoulder is much easier to digest than lamb's leg. All meats should be well cooked so that they are light and therefore easier to digest; the best way of cooking meat is boiling it slowly for a long period of time until it becomes tender. It is best to avoid rare meats. If you like fish and seafood that come from wet environments, generally they are good for the digestive system and the kidneys. The meats from animals who live on dry land are more beneficial for relieving disorders related to *Loong* and *Bad-Kan*.

3) OIL

Oil includes butter, mustard oil, sesame oil, bone marrow oil and lard. Oils help to lubricate our bodily system both internally and externally. They are good for *Loong*, impotency, massage and relaxation.

- Butter – butter is the essence of milk. It is good for virility, complexion, the digestive system and healing wounds. I always advise my patients to eat butter rather than margarine.
- Melted butter – melted butter is good for improving memory; it prolongs life and aids vision.
- Mustard oil – it has warm potency and it pacifies *Loong*; however, if it is used too much it will increase *mKhris-pa*.
- Sesame oil – it has a sharp potency, it is good for people who are under-weight and it is also good for the flexibility of the joints.

4) VEGETABLES, FRUITS AND SPICES

Vegetables

The best vegetables to eat are the ones which are available seasonally and which are locally grown, rather than ones which are frozen and transported thousands of miles from different parts of the world. Vegetables are light and easy to digest.

- Nettles – this vegetable is very well known in Tibet and it is called *sa vo*. It is closely associated with Tibet's famous yogi Milarepa who depended solely on nettles during the later stages of his long meditative retreats in the caves of Tibet. Once, when Milarepa was meditating, a few local hunters stopped at his cave to cook a meal. He gave them some nettles to cook and when they asked for salt and meat to flavour the nettle soup he simply gave them more nettles. When the hunters exclaimed that nettles were not salt and meat, Milarepa merely told them that nettles were what he used for everything. Of course it was due to his profound meditative realization that he was able to survive on just this vegetable, and Milarepa is one of the few examples of meditators who have attained enlightenment in a single lifetime. Nettles help to increase bodily heat and pacify *Loong*.

- Turnip – eliminates food poisons and toxic foods and it also helps combat altitude sickness.
- Radish – helps improve the digestive system, the gall bladder and liver, it stops diarrhoea and it pacifies *Loong*.
- Potato – clears constipation and helps anaemia; however it is not good for arthritis or for the kidneys.
- Carrot – helps strengthen the liver and eyesight.
- Rhubarb – helps kidneys and water retention.
- Yam – beneficial for menopause and energy.
- Spinach – helps constipation and anaemia.
- Cabbage – helps relieve stomach ulcers but it is not good for kidneys and arthritis.
- Beetroot – good for anaemia, osteoporosis and increases energy.
- Asparagus – strengthens the kidneys, aids water retention and rejuvenation. It is not good for gout.
- Dandelion – eliminates fever.
- Tomatoes – help blood pressure and fluid retention but are not good for arthritis.
- Onion – good for appetite and blood circulation, reduces cholesterol and pacifies *Loong* and *Bad-Kan*.
- Garlic – it has hot potency and it is good for eliminating micro-organisms, helps increase bodily heat and it is good for insomnia and increasing appetite. Too much consumption of garlic is harmful for the eyesight and liver.

- Ginger – helps blood circulation, improves bodily heat and appetite, and prevents nausea.
- Chilli – chillies are a warm potency food and good for the digestive system, bodily heat and appetite; however too much chilli can damage the lungs and liver.

Spices

A lot of traditional food in this country is quite bland and therefore it is good to add spices to your cooking to aid digestion, reduce cholesterol and also of course to improve the taste.

- Turmeric – this spice not only helps the colouring of food but also helps combat food poisoning and is good for diabetes.
- Nutmeg – alleviates heart disease and helps insomnia.
- Clove – helps nerve disorders, increases appetite, strengthens the liver and digestive system.
- Cardamom – helps kidney disorders and the digestive system.
- Cubeb – strengthens the spleen and digestive system.
- Saffron – stops bleeding and liver disorders.
- Cumin – alleviates lung infections.
- Coriander – reduces fever and helps digestion.
- Long pepper – helps asthma and cold diseases.
- Cinnamon – extracts pus from the lungs, stops diarrhoea and helps circulation of the blood.
- Asafoetida – helps heart disease, it is connected with *Loong* and eliminates micro-organisms.
- Tibetan black pepper (*yer ma*) – helps blood detoxification, clears the channels.
- Salt – gives taste to food, it is a mild laxative and gives heat.

Fruit

Fruit is a great source of natural sugar, it is easy to digest and it is also very healthy.

- Apple – stops diarrhoea and alleviates pain in the intestines and colon.
- Grapes – strengthen the lungs and eradicate fever. Good for anaemia.
- Papaya – good for the digestive system and clears constipation.
- Mango – strengthens the kidneys and the immune system.
- Banana – heals stomach ulcers and stops diarrhoea. Good for energy. However it is best not to eat bananas if you are suffering from constipation.
- Pomegranate – helps increase the strength of digestive heat, aids appetite, kidneys and blood circulation.
- Buckthorn – helps indigestion, expectorating, reduces cholesterol and helps strengthen the liver.
- Apricot – aids hair growth and heals wounds.
- Strawberries – they are an expectorant and they also help increase libido.
- Dates – excellent for energy.

Sweets such as molasses increase libido, weight, bodily heat and are diuretics. Honey strengthens the nerves, enhances the sensory organs and helps reduce weight. The honey should be natural organic honey and not the honey produced from bees fed with sugar.

5) COOKED FOODS

Due to the climatic conditions in Tibet people always ate food which was warm and cooked. I have read recently that scientists have confirmed that cooked vegetables are more beneficial for the body as the vitamins are broken down and more easily absorbed.

DRINK

In the Tibetan medical texts drink is divided into:

- Milks
- Water
- *Chang* or alcohol.

MILKS

All milks are sweet in taste and post-digestive taste. They give energy, promote good complexion and pacify *Loong* and *mKhris-pa*. Milks strengthen the seven bodily constituents and they are good for virility; too much milk, however, can produce phlegm and disturb *Bad-Kan* disorders. Warm, fresh milk just taken from the animal is said to be like nectar, however cold raw milk is heavy and bad for *Bad-Kan* and micro-organisms. Boiled milk is much easier to digest but if it is boiled too much it is difficult to digest because it becomes too concentrated.

- Cows' milk – helps lung diseases, chronic colds, diabetes, memory and helps cure dizziness and madness. It helps the seven bodily constituents and helps to produce more mother's milk when nursing. If you have problems digesting cows' milk due to its heaviness you can dilute the milk with water so it is half-milk, half-water and then boil it.
- Goats' milk – excellent for asthma, and is helpful for blood and *mKhris-pa* disorders.
- Sheep milk – it has a warm potency and therefore pacifies *Loong;* however it can aggravate heart disease and both *mKhris-pa* and *Bad-Kan*. It is bad for asthma and micro-organisms.

- Yoghurt – the taste and post-digestive taste of yoghurt is sour. It has a cool, oily potency and it aids appetite, it eliminates *Loong* related fevers, it is also good for digestion; too much yoghurt will cause constipation.
- Buttermilk – this is an excellent drink in the hot summer, the taste is astringent and sour, its potency is light, it increases digestive heat, reduces tumours, spleen diseases, piles and aids the digestion of fats.
- Sheep yoghurt and buttermilk have a warm potency while cows' yoghurt and buttermilk are lighter with cool potency.
- Cheese – increases sperm count, aids sleep, improves bodily vigour; however too much cheese will produce mucus and lead to *Bad-Kan* disorders.

Tibetan way of making butter, yoghurt and buttermilk

First of all you have to boil the milk and let it cool until it is lukewarm, then add a little yoghurt, stir and leave the mixture in a warm place overnight. Upon checking the following morning it will have formed into a thick yoghurt, which is then placed in a big wooden churner and churned slowly. Occasionally a little cold water is added. This will prevent the butter, which is forming inside the churner, from melting. After churning for approximately 40 minutes the mixture is poured into a big container in which many small lumps of yellow butter will be visible. The hands of the person making the butter should then be washed with very cold water as they now have to gather the little pieces of butter and make them into one big lump. This lump of butter is then placed into a container full of cold water, the butter is squeezed to extract the sour buttermilk; this will prevent the butter from going off.

The remaining liquid in the first container is what is known as the real buttermilk, in Tibetan known as *thara*. This *thara* can then be boiled to make fresh cheese, which is then dried with a little brown sugar added to it to make *chu-ra ngarmo* (sweet cheese). It can be dried without the sugar to make *chushii* (powdered cheese) which is then used with *tsampa* or in porridge. Tibetans also make *chu-ruu* (fungus cheese) to produce a delicious soup. In India drying the cheese can be difficult as we always have to fight with the local black crows who love the *chu-ra ngarmo*. So mirrors are placed near the cheese as it is said that the crows will be scared off by their own reflection; however I do not know if this is true or not.

I can clearly remember when I was growing up in South India, listening to my mother in the early morning, churning the yoghurt and reciting Buddhist prayers, while I lay in my bed. It is delicious to eat your own home-made butter and drink fresh buttermilk in the hot Indian summer weather.

WATER

There are seven types of water: rain, glacial, river, spring, well, sea and forest. Of these rain water is the best, like nectar, but not so much these days because of environmental pollution. In the Tibetan medical texts boiled hot water has many benefits. It helps digest fatty foods, reduces gas formation, helps asthma, colds, and flu. Cool boiled water also helps to reduce excess thirst but it should be left for at least a day.

CHANG OR ALCOHOL

Alcohol in Tibet is made from fermented wheat, barley, millet and rice and it is called *chang*. The taste is sour and bitter and when drunk it may cause diarrhoea, it increases bodily heat and sleepiness, and people become more confident and relaxed. However drinking too much can cause problems. In Tibetan medicine drunkenness has three stages. First, people become more talkative and their behaviour changes; a Tibetan proverb says that alcohol is the key for unlocking a shy person's mouth, and during this stage there is a lack of conscience and general shamelessness. The second stage is the most dangerous stage, when people start fighting, crying, and harming others. This stage is compared to a mad elephant. The third stage is when people are so drunk they are unable to remember anything. Therefore it is very important to drink in the right quantity.

THE SIX PRIMARY TASTES

All the above foods and drinks can be divided into six primary tastes and these primary tastes are generated by the five elements. When the six primary tastes are digested and absorbed by our digestive system there are three post-digestive tastes.

Relationship between the five elements, six primary tastes and three post-digestive tastes

Five Elements	Six Primary Tastes	Three Post-Digestive Tastes
Earth and water generate	Sweet taste (*mNgar-ba*)	Sweet
Earth and fire generate	Sour taste (*sKyur-ba*)	Sour
Water and fire	Salty taste (*Lan-tsha*)	Sweet
Water and air generate	Bitter taste (*Kha-ba*)	Bitter
Fire and air generate	Pungent taste (*Tsha-ba*)	Bitter
Earth and air generate	Astringent taste (*bsKa-ba*)	Bitter

For the proper functioning of mind and body we need to have the six primary tastes in our food and drink in moderate quantities, otherwise if we eat too much or too little the three principal energies will become unbalanced.

1) FOODS WITH SWEET TASTE

- Brown sugar
- Molasses
- Honey
- Potatoes
- Carrots
- Sweet potatoes
- Chocolate
- Cake
- Sweet drinks
- Milk
- Cereals
- Meat
- Grapes
- Melon
- Banana
- Turnips
- Swede

If taken in moderate quantities sweet taste is the most nutritious among the six primary tastes; it helps energy, complexion, weight increase if you are underweight, children's growth, it is an energizer if you are old, soothes the throat, heals wounds, promotes the sensory organs, aids rejuvenation, strengthens the seven bodily constituents, it is an antidote and it pacifies *Loong* and *mKhris-pa* disorders.

When taken in excess it causes obesity, diabetes, thyroid problems, urinary infections, tooth decay, parasites, sinus problems, it slows down circulation, and aggravates *Bad-Kan* related disorders. People in the West consume too much sugar and therefore problems related to excess sugar are very common.

2) FOODS WITH SOUR TASTE

- Lemon
- Lime
- Tomatoes
- Blackcurrants
- Cranberries
- Raspberries
- Strawberries
- Oranges

- Gooseberries
- Pineapple
- Blackberries
- Blueberries
- Yoghurt
- Cheese
- Pickles
- Vinegar

In moderate quantities sour taste increases appetite, aids digestion and absorption, promotes blood circulation, and clears the flow of *Loong*.

Excess sour taste causes skin problems such as boils, erysipelas, pruritus and eczema; weakening of the muscles, bones, ligaments; blurred vision, vertigo and oedema; excess thirst; aggravates infections; it causes blood disorders and problems related to *mKhris-pa*.

3) FOODS WITH SALT TASTE

- Salt
- Crisps
- Peanuts
- Savouries
- Sausages
- Ham
- Bacon
- Smoked fish
- Seaweed
- Breakfast cereals e.g. corn flakes
- Tinned food e.g. soups

When taken in moderate quantities salt taste is a laxative, it loosens the stiffness of the muscles and joints, improves circulation and gives taste to the food we eat. However a lot of our food is too highly salted and we do not need to have as much salt as they often contain.

Excess salt taste causes alopecia (baldness), premature white hair and wrinkles; dehydration, excess thirst; osteoporosis (brittle bones), weakening of energy; skin diseases; *mKhris-pa* and blood related diseases.

4) FOODS WITH BITTER TASTE

- Coffee
- Tea
- Spinach
- Broccoli
- Sour gourd
- Rhubarb
- Watercress
- Lettuce
- Asparagus
- Cabbage
- Pak choi

In moderate quantities bitter taste improves appetite, it is an antidote, it relieves thirst, cures infectious diseases, stops diarrhoea, helps reduce weight, helps hoarseness and breast diseases, and pacifies *mKhris-pa*.

Bitter taste taken in excess – such as having 10 cups of coffee and tea a day – can cause insomnia, anxiety, a weakening of the seven bodily constituents, and can disturb *Loong* and *Bad-Kan* disorders.

5) FOODS WITH PUNGENT TASTE

- Chilli
- Garlic
- Onion
- Ginger
- Radish
- Leek
- Nutmeg
- Black pepper
- Long pepper
- Asafoetida
- Whisky

In moderate quantity pungent taste helps bodily circulation and bodily heat, it aids digestion, reduces cellulite, eliminates toxins from our body, clears blockages in the channels, helps oedema and clears up skin problems.

Excess pungent taste weakens the whole of the immune system, causes ulcers, shivering, fainting, back and hip pains, bodily contraction and lowers the production of semen.

6) FOODS WITH ASTRINGENT TASTE

- Grapefruit
- Turmeric
- Buttermilk
- Courgettes
- Dandelion

In moderate quantity astringent taste heals wounds, clears complexion, reduces cellulite. However, excess astringent taste causes constipation, excess mucus production, flatulence, heart diseases and blocks the channels.

- **Sweet, sour and salty tastes pacify *Loong*.**
- **Bitter, sweet and astringent tastes pacify *mKhris-pa*.**
- **Pungent, sour and salty tastes pacify *Bad-Kan*.**

CONSUMPTION OF FOOD IN THE RIGHT QUANTITY

To consume food in moderate quantity is essential. It depends on the consistency of the food, for example if it is a heavy food you are eating – such as lamb – it is best to fill only half of your stomach. However, if it is a light food such as rice you can fill yourself up more. Your stomach must feel comfortable for the food to be easily digested. It is important to visualize your stomach in four parts: two parts for solid food, a third part for liquids and a fourth part for space. It is also important to take liquid after eating, and if you suffer from indigestion take hot boiling water.

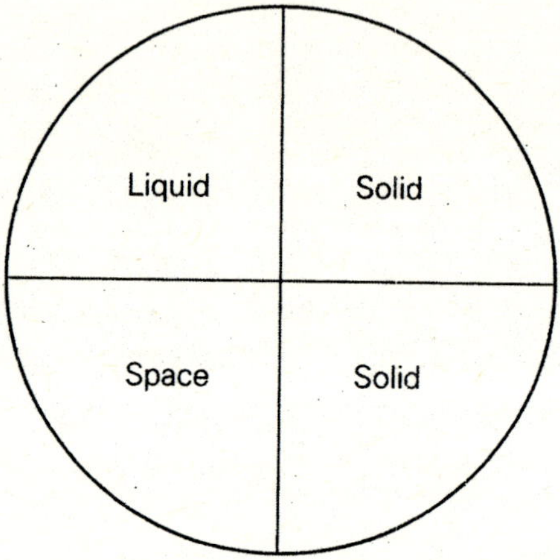

Stomach parts

Over-eating leads to an increase of mucus in the stomach which can block the channels and disturb the above digestive process; it causes all digestive illnesses. It is therefore very important to eat sensibly.

DIETARY RESTRICTIONS COVERING FOOD POISONS AND INCOMPATIBLE FOODS

Poisonous food is detected by unnatural taste and colour. If the poisonous food is burnt the smoke which appears will be as blue as a peacock's neck and the flame does not go upwards but sways to one side. If it is deliberate the poisoner will look nervous, restless and will be sweating. Poisonous food should be buried underground after it has been detected.

Incompatible foods can also harm us. For example, chicken and yoghurt, fish and milk, milk and fruit – all these are incompatible foods and when taken together they might lead to digestive problems. When taking new food which you have not tasted before it is best to take a little in the beginning in order to allow your body to become used to it.

ADVICE ON CONDUCT

This is divided into:

1 Daily conduct
2 Seasonal conduct
3 Occasional conduct

1) DAILY CONDUCT

The Tibetan medical texts teach us to spend quality time engaging in spiritual practice and to ensure we do not commit any of the 10 non-virtuous actions laid out in Buddhist teachings.

We can divide these 10 non-virtuous actions into three physical, four verbal and three mental non-virtuous actions. The 10 non-virtuous actions are:

TAKING OF LIFE

Any being who is breathing and moving has life and therefore should not be killed. We all wish to enjoy happiness and avoid suffering, and even an ant has the same feelings of self-preservation as creatures like ourselves. Being Buddhists, all Tibetans believe in rebirth and it is quite possible for an animal in this life to have been our mother in a previous life. Therefore when we remember how grateful we are to our parents in this life, we should treat all beings as our parents and therefore with respect. Having been brought up in a Tibetan community I can appreciate the good influence of the Buddhist teachings on the younger people. It is quite common for a child to try to save an insect which they see crawling on the main road. It is natural for them to say *'Nying-je'* which is a common Tibetan expression of compassion. I have been very impressed by people in this country who are great animal lovers. However, we have to remember that creatures such as spiders also have the same feelings as our pets and therefore should not be looked upon as horrible and killed.

ADULTERY

The relationship between partners, whether they are husband and wife or not, should not simply be based on sexual needs but also on mutual respect and understanding. It is very important for people to have good communication between each other and to talk openly about what sort of problems they face in their relationship. We must realize that we all have weaknesses and that nobody is perfect, and it is best if we appreciate the positive qualities which we have rather than always focusing on the negative. A person who criticizes their partner over the slightest thing and who is constantly nagging them will not be taken seriously. Nagging is the last thing people want to hear after a hard day's work.

If you see a fault in your partner it is much more effective to tell them in a relaxed atmosphere rather than moaning at them as soon as they walk in through the door. We all like to be appreciated by others and if, for example, you are a husband who is working it is a good gesture to buy flowers for your wife and to go out for dinner once in a while to show her how important she is to you. Similarly if you are a housewife looking after children it is good to realize that it is one of the important jobs in life. Tibetans consider the mother to be the person who makes peace and harmony within the family, therefore it is very good to show love and care not only to the children but also to the husband.

If there is a loving atmosphere at home the relationship will be strong, otherwise if there is too much criticism and neglect it might affect the relationship. During this time both partners feel lonely and vulnerable and if there is another person who shows them love and appreciation an affair might easily begin. Once this becomes known by the other partner and by the children it will break up all family harmony and stability. This in turn is very damaging for the young children and it will affect them for the rest of their lives. From meeting patients, I have seen a lot of young women whose fathers have had an affair and this has then affected their own relationships in a very negative way.

Susan, who is in her early thirties, told me that she can not trust any man. When she was a child she worshipped her father and when she discovered he was having an affair she was devastated. Since then she has been unable to trust any man and it now affects her own relationships with men. Whenever she begins a relationship she immediately has a fear of losing her partner and this makes her very suspicious and accusatory; she always wants to know their slightest movement and she becomes obsessed by it. Naturally this constant suspicion and mistrust makes her new partner feel suffocated and the relationship breaks down.

When talking with her I gave her the example that on her hand her five fingers were all different although they belonged to the same hand; like this all men are not the same and that many of them are good and decent. The important thing for Susan was to learn how to trust people. I told her that if she was accused of being a thief by her neighbour when she had never set foot in their house, she would be very angry and upset. Yet this was exactly what she was doing in her own relationships. She would have to slowly learn how to trust men, in the same way that we test the depth of water by going in slowly and carefully.

The above example can equally apply to a son who is traumatized by his mother having an affair when he is growing up. It is true to say that a lot of people from broken marriages lose their family roots and often have no connection with close relatives such as their grandparents, cousins and even their brothers and sisters. Therefore if your relationship is in difficulty it is best to try all means possible to save it; if this is not possible then it is best to part as peacefully as possible, especially if there are children involved.

STEALING

This simply means taking what is not yours and what has not been given to you. When I read in the papers or see on the television young people stealing from old and frail pensioners it makes me feel very sad. If we are young it is important to realize that one day we too will become old and vulnerable. His Holiness the Dalai Lama says that if you can not help people at least do not harm them, and stealing is obviously a form of great harm and in some cases can lead to worse actions such as killing.

LYING

This simply means not telling the truth and it includes all the white lies which we tell every day. Things often start from a small white lie and before we know it we have gone on to bigger things, with the truth becoming more and more obscured. Speaking truthfully and openly might be painful at times but it is therapeutic and there is no fear of leaving things covered up. The Tibetans have a saying that if your lies are as strong as iron, sooner or later the iron will melt. If we continually tell lies we will eventually lose our friends and the trust of our family.

GOSSIPING

Some people enjoy interfering with other people's lives and this kind of behaviour can be very irritating for others and tiring for yourself if you are the instigator. Before talking about others it is best to check the facts, otherwise spreading unfounded rumours will only bring trouble upon yourself. In today's society there are cases of people being sued for this wrong form of action and losing large amounts of money to say nothing of their reputation.

VERBAL ABUSE

Everyone likes a little praise and appreciation, and no one will reject being praised reasonably. However, if you praise someone too much it can sound artificial. If you abuse someone by making sarcastic remarks and picking up on their slightest faults this can cause mental distress. This can especially be the case at school when children are abused by others, or at home by their parents. In these circumstances it is easy for children to lose their self-esteem and to feel rejected.

Carol, who is in her mid-twenties, came to see me to have treatment for her mouth ulcers and gynaecological problems. She has been responding well to the treatment, but when she came for her first consultation I read her pulse and performed urinalysis, which were very much *Loong* nature – this indicated a deep suppression of her emotions. In order to build her trust I did not mention this to her immediately. When she came for a second visit I advised her that she needed to relax more, and in response to this she told me that she did not know how to relax. I asked about her childhood and whether it was happy or not, and at this point she broke down and began to cry. She told me she was sexually abused by her uncle and verbally abused by her parents who did not believe her when she told them about it. The reaction of her parents had a devastating effect on her and robbed her of her confidence in life. As she is an only child she had no one to turn to.

Her parents criticized her constantly, telling her that whatever she did was not good enough, insisting that she did everything in the way they wanted. In the family house she was not allowed to change a single piece of furniture, except in her bedroom. Because the family was isolated and did not have much contact with others, such as inviting friends for a meal, she had to suppress her feelings over many years. Eventually she moved away from her parents and got married, despite the threats of her parents to disown her because they did not agree with her choice of husband. She now had her own house, but still she was unable to do things in her own way without the fear of being criticized, due to the strong influence of her parents and their constant verbal abuse. When she called them they were dismissive and still critical of her, telling her only to call them when she had something important to tell them. She was also nervous and petrified of making mistakes in cooking or conversation, for example, when her husband invited his friends to their house for a meal.

When telling me all of this Carol cried for an hour and I listened to her as sympathetically as possible. I felt that it was very good for her to bring out all of her pain and anguish which she had been storing inside herself for so many years. I advised her not to be so afraid of her parents as she was now leading an independent life, and that we all have weaknesses so she should not be too harsh on herself when she makes mistakes. She should now enjoy her life as she has met a wonderful husband who is supportive and caring, and that she should have no fear of doing whatever she wanted in her own home. With regard to her parents I advised her that she should keep a bit of distance and not to call them so often in order to stop them from still trying control her life. This is a real-life example of the negativity which can be caused by malicious speech.

DIVISIVE SPEECH

In Tibetan this is called having two tongues and this is the same in English as calling someone two-faced. One thing is said to a person's face which might be nice, and then another thing is said to their back, which might be not so nice. If there are two close friends and you go and tell each one a different story, you might cause conflict and break their friendship. On a larger scale politicians can do this and create a war between two countries.

COVETOUSNESS

This means desiring something which belongs to somebody else and making a great effort to get it. It is a form of obsession and stems from feelings of jealousy and envy. Seeking these kind of goals could lead to any form of negative action being committed in order to achieve them.

HARMFUL INTENT

Some people do have evil thoughts and wish bad things to happen to others or can have feelings of joy over other people's pain and suffering. It can mean plotting the destruction of someone's life by calculating, pre-meditating and waiting for a long time before performing any kind of action. If you are near such a person who has harmful intent it is possible that their negative energy will make you feel very uncomfortable and you will wish to leave their presence.

ERRONEOUS VIEWS

This is to do with faith and religion. Whether to believe in religion or not is your choice, but do not criticize others for their views. I have met many patients who have changed their faith in recent years, for example many westerners who have become Buddhists, and this has often led to conflict and misunderstanding with their partners and family. I always advise people not to preach or discuss religious issues if there is no interest from others. It is far better to find some common ground where everyone can talk and enjoy the topic of conversation during a gathering of friends and family. Religion is an individual choice and preference. In addition, the medical texts detail the following things which must be considered in our daily conduct.

With regard to money, when you save, save well, and when you spend, be generous. If you win something you should know your limit. If you did something wrong admit it, be friendly with people and remember the kindness shown to you by friends and relatives; respect your parents and elders. Always try to assist those afflicted by sorrow or mental suffering, disabled people, the destitute, and beggars; never look down on those less fortunate. One should regard all beings as the same as oneself. With regard to actions, do things at the right time. With regard to sex, it is good to have as much as you desire in the winter, every two days in the spring and autumn, and once every fortnight in the summer. Too much sex can weaken the whole system, especially the eyes.

Tibetan Buddhists believe in spiritual power and meditation. We often wear blessing threads for protection and gold and diamonds to prolong life and get rid of obstacles. In the West meditation has become very fashionable. However people often begin to meditate without having a proper foundation and become disappointed when they do not get the results they desire. In Tibetan Buddhism we say, *thoo, sam, gom sum* which can be roughly translated as: learning, contemplating and meditating. So first of all we have to educate ourselves by attending lectures and teachings in the same way as bees collect the essence of many different flowers to make honey. Once we have gathered the information, we need to both study and contemplate it, just as the Buddha told people to thoroughly examine and investigate what he was saying and not simply to have blind faith. Only after this do we meditate and continue to do so on a daily basis. In order to train our mind we need patience and perseverance. Gradually we will be able to reduce negative thoughts such as anger, jealousy, selfishness and close-mindedness and increase positive thoughts such as love and compassion. Whether we become enlightened or not will not matter so much because at least we will have become a better person. A calm mind is the key to physical wellbeing.

2) SEASONAL CONDUCT

For seasonal conduct the internal five elements and the external five elements are connected, so we have to behave in accordance with the change of seasons.

Here in England winters can get extremely cold and although it can be nice and warm indoors it is very important to wear adequate clothing when going outside. When it is cold you should wear thick woollen socks and a warm hat. Once the feet are warm they can generate heat and the rest of the body warms up quickly, otherwise if you wear layer upon layer of clothes on the upper part of your body but neglect to keep your feet warm, then your body as a whole will not be warm.

If you suffer from arthritis it is important to keep the knees warm by wearing knee warmers, thick socks for the feet and gloves for the hands, also try to have hot baths with bath salts in the evenings. If you suffer from asthma it is important to keep the chest warm, people with weak kidneys need to keep their back warm by wearing long jumpers and cardigans. As a general rule I would very much advise women to wear trousers and long skirts in the winter rather short skirts. Such simple precautions can prevent colds and flu. In the winter lamb and soups are excellent warming foods, if you are vegetarian then garlic and ginger should be added to foods and soups as much as possible. A little wine or perhaps a peck of whisky in the very cold weather is also acceptable.

In spring one should eat honey and have lots of hot water, one should have food and drink such as ginger decoction, barley and beef. One should do lots of exercise and have massages with pea flour.

In the dry summer one should eat light, sweet and cooling food such as rice, beef and vegetables; avoid direct sunshine; have cool baths; drink alcohol mixed with spring water. One should wear pure cotton clothes and sandals with no socks. I see many people in the summer wearing shorts, a T-shirt but also thick socks and training shoes. This does not help you to keep cool and in the summer it is important to let your feet breathe.

Summer activities such as swimming and walking by the coast are also very good for you. It is important not to become over-exposed to the sun as our skin is not used to the sharp sunlight, which with the increase in pollution and changing climate patterns is becoming much more common. These days a lot of people are suffering from skin cancer because of over-exposure to the sun. The nature of the eyes is hot and it is therefore also very important to protect them from the strong glare of the sun by wearing good quality sunglasses. When it is very hot it is important to shower daily to avoid any skin irritations arising from excess perspiration.

Drinks such as buttermilk, fresh fruit juice and mineral water should be taken as they are healthy, cooling and refreshing. With regard to alcohol, drinking wine and spirits in excess can also be harmful as they are hot potency and they can burn the bodily system both internally and externally. Drinking a cool beer in moderation is much more acceptable. You can also eat lots of fresh fruit and vegetables, fish and beef.

In wet summer one should drink buttermilk and eat food which generates digestive heat such as garlic, ginger, cinnamon and nutmeg. In autumn one should eat sweet, bitter and astringent food, and wear clothes scented with sandalwood and camphor.

3) OCCASIONAL CONDUCT

Regarding occasional conduct one should not suppress certain natural bodily functions. In the Tibetan medical texts there are 13 natural functions of the body and they are:

- **Hunger** – when we are hungry we should eat, otherwise if we suppress our hunger by doing things such as skipping meals over a long period of time, it will lead to problems such as vertigo and anorexia. When these have arisen it is best to eat in small quantities many times a day, beginning with something light and nutritious such as hot soup.
- **Thirst** – when we suppress our thirst our bodies become dehydrated and this can lead to giddiness and diseases related to the heart, and in some extremes it can also lead to madness. To combat this one should begin by taking food and drinks with cool potency.
- **Vomiting** – we all know how horrible it is when our stomach is churning and wants to vomit. If we suppress this it will lead to headaches, breathing problems and eye diseases. The best thing is to always be sick if there is the urge, and then to fast in order to cleanse oneself.
- **Sneezing** – if we wish to sneeze and we try to stop ourselves, it will lead to stiffness in the neck, eyesight problems and headaches. In some extremes it might distort the mouth because of the disruption caused to the flow of *Loong*. To combat these problems we need nasal medication and medicated inhalations. A good sneeze will clear all of our senses.
- **Yawning** – this is very similar to sneezing and the above points also apply here.
- **Breathing** – suppression of breathing is a big problem here in the West. People's breathing is very shallow and this can lead to cardiac diseases and mental illnesses. This is

because the flow of the all pervasive *Loong* is blocked and for the normal function of heart and mind it is vital that it is allowed to flow freely. It is good to do breathing exercises and meditations which are concentrated on the breath.

- **Sleep** – this can be especially applicable to people who work unusual hours, such as night-shift workers. It can also be applicable to people who fly a lot through different time zones. I have a patient who has all the symptoms of lack of sleep mentioned in the Tibetan medical texts. The patient is continually yawning, suffers tiredness and dullness of mind, and is unable to focus their mind. To treat these symptoms one needs a full body massage, a good glass of red wine, and best of all, long undisturbed sleep.
- **Sputum (phlegm)** – when this is swallowed back instead of expectorated it will accumulate in the chest and cause breathing problems. If you need to expectorate it is best to find a quiet place and do so. If you have too much sputum it is best to avoid milk products and instead have drinks such as fresh root ginger tea.
- **Tears** – sometimes it is very therapeutic to have a good cry to release the accumulated frustration, anger, disappointment and sadness in our lives. If we suppress our emotions too much it will contribute to heart disease and loss of appetite. It is therefore important to have good friends and close family with whom you can share your sorrows and try to find a solution to your problems, rather than keeping everything inside and feeling sorry for yourself. This can be especially true for men in the West who are traditionally reserved and introvert.
- **Wind** – this can be one of the most unsociable activities to perform and it is best to do well away from other people, for example in a toilet. Suppression of wind causes flatulence, pain in the stomach and dry faeces.

- **Faeces** – these days people can be so busy they do not have time to properly eliminate the waste products from their bodies. This can create problems such as bad breath, headaches, bloated stomach, and a feeling of heaviness in mind and body. It is therefore always advisable to allow your body to function normally and once in a while something like colon irrigation is of benefit.
- **Urine** – suppression of the urine can lead to urinary and kidney stones, and other urinary diseases. It very advisable to listen to your body and to go when there is an urge to release urine.
- **Sperm** – when the release of sperm is suppressed for too long through no sexual activity it can lead to premature ejaculation, urine retention, pain in the genitals and it can also affect male potency. It therefore advisable to release sperm through sexual activity.

From the above natural bodily functions, suppression of thirst, breathing and tears can lead to heart disease and mental problems which I have found to be common in this country. These can be prevented through regular breathing exercises, drinking enough water and being more expressive.

9

TREATMENT TECHNIQUES – PART II

This second chapter of treatment looks at prescribing medicine, pharmacology and therapies.

PRESCRIBING MEDICINE

When prescribing medicine there are 10 factors to take into consideration. These are the individual body constitution of the patient, strength of the patient, age, metabolic rate, condition of the disease, location of the disease, climatic factors, time of manifestation, bodily nature and checking to see if the patient is used to taking this form of medicine. After these 10 factors have been considered we treat each patient individually. In Tibetan we say that if we do not consider all the above factors in relation to each individual case, it would be like putting the load of a yak on the back of a sheep, or a sheep's load on the back of a yak.

Written in 1717, Geshe Tenzin Phuntsok's materia medica of Tibetan medicine, called *Dri-med Shel-gong Shel-phren*, mentions 2,294 different medical substances used in Tibetan medicine. They can be all be classified within the following eight categories:

1 Precious gemstones and metals
2 Soils
3 Minerals
4 Wood
5 Mucilaginous
6 Shrubs
7 Herbs
8 Animal products

In the *rGyud-bzhi* it says that our bodies are made of five elements and the *Nyes-pa-gsum* are caused by the imbalance of the five elements. The antidotes – which are comprised of herbs and minerals – are also generated by these same five elements. Following from this the five elements generate the six primary tastes of the medicines. (See table on page 111 on advice on diet).

- Problems related to *Loong* are treated by medicines which are a combination of sweet, sour, salty and hot tastes.
- Problems related to *mKhris-pa* are treated by combinations of bitter, sweet and astringent tastes.
- Problems related to *Bad-Kan are* treated by combinations of hot, sour and salty tastes.

In Tibetan medicine most medicinal preparations are combinations of the eight potencies which are: heavy, oily, cooling, blunt, light, rough, hot and sharp. In greater detail these eight potencies can be divided into the 17 qualities which can counteract the 20 subtle natures of *Loong*, *mKhris-pa* and *Bad-Kan*.

Earth has the following qualities: heavy, stable, blunt, smooth, oily and dry. These qualities pacify *Loong* disorders because the nature of *Loong* is light, movable, cool, rough, hard and thin. Earth can also aggravate *Bad-Kan* because they share the same qualities.

Water has the following qualities: fluidity, cooling, heavy, blunt, oily and supple. These qualities pacify *mKhris-pa* disorders because the nature of *mKhris-pa* is oily, pungent, hot, light, sharp and moist. Water can also aggravate *Bad-Kan* because they share the same qualities.

Fire has the following qualities: hot, sharp, dry, coarse, light, oily and mobile. These qualities pacify *Bad-Kan* disorders because the nature of *Bad-Kan* is cool, blunt, smooth, sticky, heavy, steady and oily. Fire can aggravate *mKhris-pa* because they share the same qualities.

Air has the following qualities: light, mobile, cold, coarse, pale and dry. These qualities pacify *Bad-Kan* disorders. Air can aggravate *Loong* because they share the same qualities.

1) PRECIOUS GEMSTONES AND METALS

Below are examples of some of the precious gemstones and metals which are used in Tibetan medicine.

Gemstones

Name	Taste	Potency	Uses
Pearl	Astringent	Cool	Treats brain damage due to injury or inflammation; nerve degeneration; stiffness and contraction of the tendons and ligaments; paralysis. Is an antidote.
Coral	Astringent	Cool	Treats hepatitis; inflammation of the nerves. Is an antidote.
Lapis	Astringent	Cool	Treats skin diseases; relieves itching; helps prevent premature greying of the hair. It is an antidote.
Ruby	Astringent	Cool	Balances the *Nyes-pa-gsum* and dispels evil spirits.

Sapphire	Astringent	Cool	It is a panacea and therefore helps all kinds of diseases.
Emerald	Astringent	Cool	Reduces fever, helps epilepsy and neurological diseases.
Turquoise	Astringent	Cool	Treats eye diseases and hepatitis. It is an antidote.
GZi (black & white striped stone unique to Tibet)	Astringent	Cool	Treats epilepsy, cures diseases and headaches.
Achates	Astringent	Cool	Treats epilepsy, eye diseases and headaches.

Metals

Gold (24 carat)	Astringent	Cool	Treats oxide poison, prolongs life, aids rejuvenation.
Silver	Astringent	Cool	Treats arthritis, lymph diseases, dried pus and impure blood.
Copper	Sweet	Cool	Treats hepatitis, inflammation of the lungs
Iron	Astringent	Cool	Treats oedema, eye diseases, eliminates toxins from the liver.

In the process of preparation all gems and metals have to be detoxified, refined and powdered before they can be used as medicine, otherwise they will have an adverse effect.

2) SOILS

Below are some of the different soils used in Tibetan medicine.

Name	Taste	Potency	Uses
Yellow Sulphur	Astringent	Neutral	Expels evil spirits, heals wounds and infections
Natron	Sweet and salty	Hot	Treats indigestion, tumours, micro-organisms. It is an antidote.
Yellow Ochre	Sweet	Cool	Treats inflammation of the nerves and five vital organs, burns, wounds and infections.

3) MINERALS

Below are some of the minerals which are used in Tibetan medicine.

Name	Taste	Potency	Uses
Orpiment	Bitter	Hot	Treats glandular fever and septic wounds.
Calamine	Astringent	Cool	Treats hepatitis, heals bone cracks and fractures.
Stalactite	Astringent	Hot	Heals tendons and ligaments damaged through injury.
Magnet	Astringent	Hot	Removes iron nails and bullets from the body, heals cracks and bone fractures, aids cranial nerve disorders.
Calcite	Sweet	Hot	Treats ulcers, heartburn, diarrhoea, eliminates fever, heals cracked bones and fractures.

All soils and minerals are detoxified and incinerated before being powdered and used as medication.

The following ingredients – **wood, mucilaginous, shrubs** and **herbs** – used in the preparation of Tibetan medicine have to follow the seven important procedures. These are:

THE PLANTS SHOULD GROW IN THEIR OWN NATURAL HABITAT

For example, a cool potency medicine such as gentian should grow in a cold climate like Tibet, and a hot potency medicine such as pomegranate should grow in a hot climate like India. The surroundings of where the plants are grown should be clean, spacious and have good light; plants grown in these surroundings should also be healthy, undamaged by insects and the weather. It is considered bad to pick plants grown near places such as cemeteries or places of refuse.

THE PLANTS SHOULD BE COLLECTED AT THE RIGHT TIME

Different plants grow in different seasons, and all the different parts of the plant should be collected at the appropriate time.

Root plants such as dandelion, rhubarb, solomon's seal, rheum nobile; the stem parts such as moonseed, blackberry; the trunk parts such as eaglewood, white and red sandalwood – should all be collected in the late autumn as this is the time when the plants are their most potent and all the plant nutrients are stored in those particular parts.

Leaf parts of the plants such as halerpestes sarmentosa, phlogacanthus pubinervius, spleenwort; the latex parts of the plant such as spurge, euphorbia royleana; the stalk parts of the plant such as horned cumin – should all be collected in the wet summer as this is the time when these parts are at their peak potency.

Flower parts of the plants such as wild rose, rhododendron arboreaum, yellow and pink lousewort; the fruit parts of the plant such as emblica officinalis, pomegranate, nutmeg; the seed parts of the plant such as caraway, anemone rivularis – should be collected when they are fully ripened in the middle of the autumn when they at their most potent.

Bark parts of the plants such as northern ash, cinnamon, China berry; inner-rind parts of the plants such as barberry, rosehip; sap such as saps from pine and sal trees – should all be collected in the spring when the plants are at the peak energy and at their most potent.

Plants with a **purgative potency** such as croton, liburnum and chickweed – should be collected at the end of the autumn when the water and earth elements are at their peak and have been absorbed by the roots.

Plants with an **emetic potency** such as inkberry, thistle and sweetflag – should be collected in the early spring when the plant buds are first appearing and the fire and air elements are at their peak strength.

According to the lunar calendar the plants are collected when the moon is waxing. When being collected Medicine Buddha mantras are recited.

DETOXIFICATION

This involves the separation of the toxic parts of the plant; after the plants have been collected their toxic parts have to be eliminated. These toxic parts will not cause death, however, they are removed in order to protect our digestive system, seven bodily constituents and subtle flow of *Loong* energy.

Plant Part	Toxic parts to be removed
Roots	Outer skin
Trunk	Inner rind
Stem	Stem joints
Leaves	Leaf stalks
Flowers	Sepal
Latex	Heat unsalted butter, add latex and simmer slowly. Toxins are released through the vapours.
Sap	No need to detoxify
Seeds	No need to detoxify
Bark	Scratch the outer layer

SORTING AND DRYING

When I was a student at the Tibetan and Astrological Institute it was part of our studies to go to Manali in Himachal Pradesh every September for herbs collection. This area in the Himalayas is very close to Tibet and a lot of the plants which grow in Tibet can also be found there. It was very moving and sad for us to know that our own country was so close to where we were. As most of us had been born in India, our second home, Tibet was a place to which we had never been. A Tibetan medical professor would take us and introduce us to each and every individual plant, its name, taste, potency and usage. It was a wild and beautiful place with glacial valleys, natural waterfalls and sheep roaming freely, and sometimes we would be in competition with the sheep to get to the same plant!

We would get up early in the morning and return in the evening, spending the whole day collecting herbs. We would then wash the roots of the plants in the local water which was so cold that while washing the roots we had to stop for short periods because we could not feel our hands. Once they had been washed all the different parts of the plant had to be separately sorted and allowed to dry. If the plant was cool potency it was dried in cool air and shade, if it was hot potency it was dried in the sun and fire. Any potential pollutants nearby would affect the potency of the plants and therefore were avoided.

DURATION AND POTENCY

For maximum potency, medicines should contain plants which were picked in the same year. The older the plant the less potency it has and therefore its healing effect will not be so great.

FOLLOW PHARMACOLOGICAL PROTOCOL

Pharmacological formula make the plants easier to ingest and assimilate, as does compounding of ingredients for proper usage according to the pharmacological texts.

4) WOOD MEDICATIONS

Wood medications are compounded from roots, tree trunks, stems, bark, sap, leaves, flowers and fruit. Examples are:

Eaglewood – helps relieve heart fevers and life-channel.
White sandalwood – eliminates agitated fevers of the lungs and heart.
Red sandalwood – eliminates blood fevers.
Frankincense – subdues demonic influences and acts as an analgesic.
Birthwort – relieves fevers of the blood and blood diseases.

5) MUCILAGINOUS

These are plant essences. For example, camphor eliminates acute and chronic fevers; saffron eliminates all diseases connected to the liver and stops internal bleeding; nutmeg pacifies *Loong* and eliminates heart disease.

6) SHRUBS

The shrubs which we use in Tibetan medicine are grown on plains in a hot climate. Shrub medications are compounded of roots, stalks, leaves, flowers and fruit. Examples of shrubs are acacia which is used to treat arthritis and reduce inflammation and skin diseases; barberry helps arrest poisons in the body and drains the lymphs; felwort treats jaundice; liquorice treats lung disease and nerve disorders; liburnum treats liver disorders and is a laxative; raspberry treats epidemics; elecampane treats flatulence, gas formation, ulcers, diphtheria and heals wounds.

7) HERBS

Tibet is called *Men-Jong,* the land of medicine. Before the Chinese invaded Tibet in 1950 there were over 300 species of medicinal plants which grew in Tibet and their supply was plentiful. However, when a survey was conducted in 1990 many were found to be extinct including white sedum, frittillaria, codonopsis nervosa, angelica and panax pseudo. The remaining medicinal plants were also found to be in greatly reduced amounts of supply. This was especially the case for the Kongpo region of Tibet and Lhamo Lhatso (the sacred lake where the birth place of the Fourteenth Dalai Lama was foreseen). In these places many Chinese come to stay for three months and take a powerful medicinal plant tonic called *ya-tsa-gun-bu* (summer grass-winter worm). In Eastern Tibet from an area in Kham – called *Kye-gu-Dho* – 176,785 kilos of this tonic has been exported by the Chinese and in the Tibetan

Autonomous Region since 1962 122,850 kilos of frittillary has been taken.

Between 1958 and 1966 in the Kham area of *Balung Zong* the Chinese took over one million kilos of medicinal plants including wickweed (sheep's jaw), heracleum lallii root and codonopsis nervosa. All of these plants were dug up from the roots with no programme of replanting. These actions by the Chinese have had a very destructive effect on the Tibetan environment and on the future supply of Tibetan herbal medicine.

- Lagotis grass helps to alleviate fevers of the solid viscera, turbid fever and rigidity of the thighs caused by *Loong* disorders.
- Tibetan primula cures contagious poisons and chronic fevers.
- Nodding dragon head alleviates fevers in the stomach and hepatitis.
- White gentian alleviates sore throat and fevers caused by poisons.
- Frittillaria heals fractures of the skull and alleviates fevers caused by poisoning.
- Bluethorn poppy heals fractured bones, alleviates fevers of the bones and strengthens cancellate bone.
- Angelica alleviates fever in the heart and poisoning.
- The flowers and fruit of barberries cure diarrhoea.
- Henbane alleviates worms.
- Carex alleviates eye diseases and strengthens the eyes. It is also a remedy for wounds of the trunk.
- Catnip removes albugo from the cornea.
- Policeman's helmet regulates heavy periods.
- Tansy stops haemorrhages, reduces water retention of the limbs, kidney disease and has rejuvenating properties.
- Lakeweed alleviates serums and dropsy.

- Marshmallow alleviates urine retention, fever of the kidneys and diarrhoea.
- Withlow grass cures meat poisons.
- Shepherd's purse cures vomiting.
- Orchid is a tonic and it increases sperm count.
- Caltrops alleviates water retention, arthritis and kidney disease.
- Columbine removes foreign bodies such as an arrowhead or a dead embryo.
- Strawberry extracts blood, pus and serum.
- Cumin treats eye disease, poisoning and fever caused by *Loong* disorders.
- Sweet clover and valerian cure chronic fever and fever caused by poisons.
- Larkspur treats diarrhoea.
- Pennycress treats coughs and kidney infections.
- Spurge treats both hot and cold diseases and is used as an emetic.
- Hog's fennel treats serum, cold kidney disorders and lumbar problems.
- Solomon's seal promotes longevity and treats serum.
- Four o'clock root increases male potency, strengthens the kidneys and dries up serums.
- Burweed alleviates contagious poison and kidney infection and fever caused by trauma.
- Indian madder treats pulmonary and renal diseases.
- Tamarisk and male fern treat meat poison and compounded poison.
- Knotweed treats fever of the hollow organs and the small and large intestines.
- Tibetan lancea strengthens the lungs and extracts pus from the lungs.

8) ANIMAL PRODUCTS

In the Tibetan medical texts various kinds of animal products are mentioned, however few are used. As Buddhists, Tibetans try to avoid killing other living beings.

- Fish strengthen the eyesight, appetite, heal wounds, dissolve tumours and strengthen the digestive system.
- Sheep's brain treats vertigo.
- Goat's brain heals tendons and ligaments.
- Goat's liver is a tonic for the eyes.
- Otter's liver treats urine retention.
- Goat's heart treats worms.
- Rabbit's heart treats angina, madness and demonic possession.
- Sheep's bone treats *Loong* disorders.
- Pig's bone alleviates stomach ulcers.
- Musk treats worms, inflammation, poisons and kidneys.
- Bezoar treats contagious poison, fever of the liver and hollow viscera.
- Pig's fat treats skin diseases, gathers poisons together, promotes hair growth.
- Snake skin treats lucoderma and eczema.
- Wild Yak's horn dissolves tumours and improves bodily heat.

PHARMACOLOGY

When treating the patient Tibetan medicine does not suppress the disease. Whatever disease has spread to our five vital organs, six hollow organs and seven bodily constituents first has to be arrested by giving medicine in the form of decoction. If the disease is deep within us, such as in our muscles or bones, it has to be aggravated in order to be brought out and during this period the patient will feel a lot worse due to the decoction. It is very common for my patients to contact me after a week of first taking their medicine and telling me that they feel worse. I tell them that this is a very good sign, that the medicine is having an effect and that they should continue taking it. After continuing for a month the patients then tell me they are feeling better. If the disease is stagnant in our body, for example if it is a tumour, it has to be brought out by prescribing a long-term course of pill medicine to dissolve the tumour. When going through the treatment process it is natural to feel some discomfort and pain. If we have a thorn in our finger to remove it will be painful, but it is impossible to get it out without digging into our skin and therefore causing pain.

TEN DIFFERENT FORMS OF MEDICINES

From the eight classifications of the medicinal ingredients listed in the medical texts, the following 10 different forms of medicines can be prepared:

1 Decoction (*Thang*)
2 Powder (*Phye-ma*)
3 Pills (*Ril-bu*)
4 Medicinal paste (*lDe-gu*)
5 Medicinal butter (*sMan-mar*)
6 Medicinal ash (*Thal-snan*)
7 Concentrated decoction (*Khan-dra*)
8 Medicinal wine (*sMan-chang*)
9 Gem medicine compounds (*Rin-po-che*)
10 Herbal compounds (*sNgo-sbyor*)

These days the most common form of Tibetan medicine is in pill form as it is compact, easy to count, easy to take, and easy to carry.

1) DECOCTION

The advantage of taking medicine in the form of decoction is that the ingredients are absorbed quickly after ingestion and they immediately take effect. There are 55 different combinations of decoctions mentioned in the Tibetan medical texts and here I will give four examples, listing their composition and their use and action.

- **Elecampane 4** (*Ma-Nu-bZhi-Thang*)
  Composition – elecampane, moonseed, blackberry, ginger.
  Use & Action – it is taken in the beginning stages of influenza when the symptoms are cold chills, headaches and joint pains. It reduces sweat and balances the body temperature.
- **Tribulus 3** (*gZe-Ma-gSum-Thang*)
  Composition – caltrop, Tibetan marsh mallow, crab.
  Use & Action – it is diuretic and it eliminates kidney diseases.
- **Quince 4** (*Tahr-bhoo-bZhi-Thang*)
  Composition – quince, sumach, oak powder, barberry flower, buttermilk.
  Use & Action – stops diarrhoea.
- **Moonseed 3** (*Lay-Tay-gSum-Thang*)
  Composition – moonseed, mineral pitch, myrobalam.
  Use & Action – treats gout.

Dosage

Mix a tablespoon of herbs with three glasses of water, bring it to the boil and then let it simmer gently until one-third of the liquid is remaining. The decoction is strained through a cheese cloth or a tea strainer and allowed to cool a little. When it is warm it can be drunk at the times instructed by the physician.

2) POWDER

When a decoction is not strong enough, medicine in powder form is used. In the Tibetan medical texts 170 different kinds of powder medicines are listed; powder medicine is often made into pill form. Here I will give two examples of powder medicine, along with their composition, use and action.

- **Pomegranate 5** *(Se-bru 5)*
  Composition – pomegranate, piper longum, cardamom, cinnamon, liburnum.
  Use & Action – increases digestive heat, relieves flatulence, improves blood circulation, reduces pain in the kidneys and hips.
- **Calcite 6** (*Choong-she* 6)
  Composition – calcite, pomegranate, cardamom, piper longum, elecampane, saffron.
  Use & Action – relieves acidity and heartburn, pacifies *Bad-Kan* disorders.

Dosage

Four grams taken in the morning on an empty stomach with warm water.

3) PILLS

Pill medicines are prepared through grinding all the ingredients into a fine powder; water is added for binding, the mixture is rolled into pills which can be as small as a baby pea or as large as a cherry, the pills are then are dried thoroughly. Tibetan medicinal pills can contain as little as five ingredients or as many as 157.

The effect of medicine in the form of pills is slow acting and gentle, it will take a minimum of twenty-four hours for the first effects of the medicine to show. The pills are mainly prescribed for chronic diseases which have developed slowly in our body over a long period of time before they become manifest. Therefore the course of treatment will often be a long one as the medicine has to go through the tiny capillaries in our body before it can work. These days the majority of the patients who come to see me suffer from chronic problems and diseases. In the Tibetan medical texts 22 different types of pills are mentioned and here I will describe six of them, along with their composition, use and action.

- **Garuda 5** (*Khyung-iNga*)
  Composition – myrobalan, costus, sweetflag, musk, aconite.
  Use & Action – treats tonsillitis, diphtheria, skin diseases, muscular pain, micro-organisms and is an analgesic.
- **Felwort 8** (*Tik-Ta-8*)
  Composition – felwort, snake gourd, aconite, costus, horned cumin, picrorhiza kurrooa, sow thistle, barberry bark.
  Use & Action – treats jaundice and its symptoms such as headaches, high fever, nausea, bitter taste in the mouth, yellow sclera, tongue and skin.
- **Eaglewood 8** (*Agar 8*)
  Composition – eaglewood, nutmeg, hog plum, bamboo pith, sal tree resin, costus, myrobalan, kapok's calyx.
  Use & Action – treats mental unrest, insanity, loss of speech, mammary, glandular and hepatic pains, inability to concentrate.
- **Shorea Robusta 10** (*sPos-dKar 10*)
  Composition – sal tree resins, senna, hemp, costus, phlogacanthus pubinervius, terminalia chebula, belleric myrobalan, embelic myrobalan, moonseed, rock bitumen.
  Use & Action – treats gout, arthritis, skin diseases, drains lymphs and is an anti-pruritic.

- **Gentiana 15** (*sPang-rGhan 15*)
  Composition – gentiana, black eaglewood, hog plum, white sandalwood, nutmeg, bamboo pith, sweetflag, costus, terminalia chebula, embelic myrobalan, belleric myrobalan, moonseed, phlogacanthus pubinervius, clove, liquorice.
  Use & Action – it is an expectorant, bronchodialator, it subsides coughs, treats breathlessness, hoarseness and blood in the sputum.
- **Betel Nut 28** (*Gu-Yu 28*)
  Composition – betel nut, pomegranate, cinnamon, pennycress, piper longum, cardamom, liburnum, golden sand, mango, rose apple, pongamia fruit, madder, red lac, musk, medler, yellow horse-eye bean, poppy, juniper, myrobalan, snake gourd, phlogacanthus pubinervius, caltrop, crab, nodding dragon head, mellow seed, barberry, mineral pitch, turmeric.
  Use & Action – reduces swollen testicles, treats premature ejaculation and irregular periods, leukorrhea, nephrosis.

Dosage

Three pills or one big pill according to the instructions of the physician.

HOW TO TAKE TIBETAN MEDICINE

There are three ways to take Tibetan medicine and these days 99 per cent of Tibetan medicine is in pill form. How to take the pills very much depends on the strength of one's teeth! If you have strong teeth you can simply put the pills in your mouth, sip a little warm water, crush them with your teeth and then chew, taking more warm water as you go along. If your teeth are not so strong the pills need to be soaked in a little warm water for 10 minutes and then they can be chewed in the same way as above. If you have weak teeth you need to use a garlic press to break the pills and a pestle and mortar to grind them into powder which can then be taken with warm water.

Tibetan medicine contains no artificial preservatives, flavours, or chemicals to dissolve it, therefore taking Tibetan medicine with warm water helps it to be absorbed in the stomach. The taste of the medicine is bitter and I always tell my patients not to think about the taste while taking it. It is very important that the pills are preserved in an airtight jar in order for them to retain their potency.

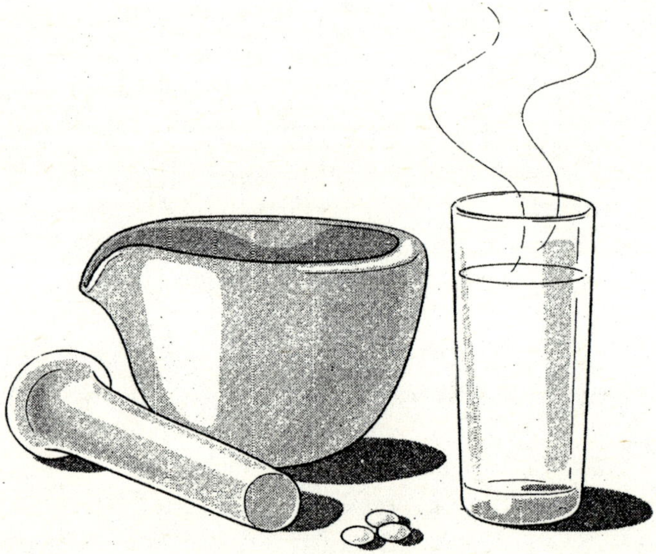

How to take Tibetan medicine

4 & 5) MEDICINAL PASTE AND MEDICINAL BUTTER

In the Tibetan medical texts 25 different types of paste medicine and 23 different types of medicinal butter are listed. However, these days their use in Tibetan medicine is not very common.

6) MEDICINAL ASH

Generally all ingredients of medicinal ash should have first been incinerated before being used as ash. For example, calcite is broken into pieces and burnt in the fire for a long time until it is completely red. This red calcite is then put into either *chang* (Tibetan alcohol) or buttermilk where it immediately dissolves and turns into a thick paste. This is dried in round shapes and then used to treat diphtheria (obstruction of the throat), tumours and chronic digestive disorders. In the medical texts 13 different types of medicinal ash are mentioned.

7) CONCENTRATED DECOCTION

The ingredients of the decoction are concentrated by being slowly boiled until they become a lump, which is dried and then used. For example, there is *brag-zhun* or common mineral pitch (in Tibetan *brag-zhun* means rock sap). This is a brownish substance found in the Himalayas as well as other mountain ranges, and it is used to treat eye disease, digestive problems, hepatitis, kidney problems, water retention and fevers caused by poisons. It is first soaked and purified in water and then filtered. The liquid is slowly boiled and stirred continuously until it has concentrated into a lump. In the medical texts 17 different concentrated decoctions are mentioned.

8) MEDICINAL WINE

In the medical texts 10 different types of medicinal wine are mentioned. Here I will give the example of barley and molasses wine.

The barley is first washed and cooked like rice and then spread on a cloth to cool. When the barley is at room temperature yeast and molasses are added; the mixture is then put in an airtight clay pot which is wrapped in a blanket in order to be kept warm. It is left for three days and after this it will smell strongly of alcohol. If it is left for a further week or two it will become fully fermented and when the pot is opened you will see a mixture which has a nice smooth consistency. A little is taken and mixed with water and left to soak for a few hours then squeezed with the hands and filtered through a cheese cloth. The residue is thrown away and the remaining liquid is drunk before going to bed. It aids sleep and relieves problems related to *Loong* disorders.

9) GEM MEDICINE

In Tibetan medicine at present, there are seven precious pills or *Rinchen Rilpo*. Four of these can only be prepared by institutions such as the Tibetan Medical and Astrological Institute in Dharamsala, the leading medical centres in Tibet, and by a very few private practitioners. This is because the gem and minerals ingredients (such as *gZi* – a precious stone unique to Tibet, one of which can cost as much as £10,000) are so expensive. Precious pills are taken if all the other forms of medicine have not worked.

The Tibetan Medical and Astrological Institute in Dharamsala is able to manufacture these medicines because a great amount of these precious gems and minerals are given by the private office of His Holiness the Dalai Lama. In Tibetan tradition, when someone dies their jewels and most precious possessions are offered to enlightened spiritual beings in order for the deceased person to accumulate good merit and achieve a good rebirth. For Tibetans His Holiness the Dalai Lama is the incarnation of Avalokiteshvara the Buddha of Compassion, and they consider it a privilege to be able to make an offering to such a being. His Holiness believes the best way in which these precious stones and minerals can be used in order to benefit others is to give them to the Tibetan Medical and Astrological Institute which can then produce the precious medicines which in turn help thousands of people. I remember as a student once seeing a container full of precious stones such as *gzhi*, coral, turquoise and pearl. It was an amazing sight to see so many precious stones together in one place.

The preparation of these precious pills can take many months as the individual ingredients have to be detoxified, incinerated and blessed. On 25th April 1982 in Dharamsala Dr Tenzin Chodrak, the senior physician to His Holiness the Dalai Lama, along with a group of 10 other Tibetan physicians and their assistants, began the preparations for making the first four precious pills listed below. It took two months for the decontamination. This was followed by the distillation and calcination of the mercury and the incineration of other ingredients such as gold, silver, iron and copper. For example, the smelting of the gold took 54 hours and the smelting of silver took 10 hours.

In Tibetan medicine purified mercury is used because it is like a panacea to treat all forms of disease especially chronic tumours; it also nourishes tissues and rejuvenates. The reason for this preparation taking such a long time was that the procedures as described in the ancient medical texts had to be followed step-by-step in order to produce the completely purified forms of these ingredients. These then had to be then compounded to produce the four precious pills. Once this had been successfully completed, religious ceremonies performed by His Holiness the Dalai Lama took place to bless and consecrate the precious pills. This was a very important occasion as it was the first time it had been done outside of Tibet since exile. Below are listed all seven precious pills used in Tibetan medicine.

- **The Great Cold Compound Precious Black Pill** (*Rinchen grang-byor Riln-Nag-Chenmo*)
  Composition – 157 different precious gems, minerals, metals and herbs. It is wrapped in an orange silk cloth.
  Use & Action – treats liver disease, ulcers, heart disease, water retention, gout, arthritis, skin diseases, food poisoning, strengthens the arteries, prevents contagious diseases. If you are healthy it can be taken for rejuvenation and to prolong one's life.
- **Precious Wish-Fulfilling Jewel** (*Rinchen Ratna Bsam-Phel*)
  Composition – 70 different precious gems, minerals, metals and herbs. It is wrapped in a light blue silk cloth.
  Use & Action – treats epilepsy, nerve disorders, paralysis, lung diseases, heart disease, incontinence, Parkinson's disease, loss of speech and memory, rigidity and contraction of the limbs, blockage of the arteries, high blood pressure, it helps in the prevention of stroke.
- **Great Multi-Compound Precious Pill** (*Rinchen Mang-Byor Chen-mo*)
  Composition – 57 different precious gems, minerals, metals and herbs. It is wrapped in a light red silk cloth.
  Use & Action – it is an antidote for poisonous bites, food chemical poisoning, stops bleeding caused by ulcers, treats hidden and chronic fevers, poor complexion, weight loss, reduces coughing and water retention. This precious pill is very popular with the Tibetan refugees who travel to large Indian cities in the winter to sell sweaters, a form of business which is one of their main sources of income. As the pill is an antidote to food poisoning and dangerous diseases such as rabies they have great faith in its effectiveness.
- **Great Purified Moon Crystal** (*Rinchen btso-bkru Da-Shel*)
  Composition – 45 different precious gems, minerals, metals and herbs. It is wrapped in a maroon silk cloth.

Use & Action – it strengthens the digestive system, treats ulcers, stomach tumours, chronic diarrhoea, hair loss, aids rejuvenation, effective for *dus-nad smug-po* which is a combination of *Loong,' mKhris-pa, Bad-Kan* and blood diseases.

- **Turquoise 25** (Rinchen Gyu-rNying 25)
  Composition – 25 minerals and herbs. It is wrapped in turquoise silk cloth.
  Use & Action – treats chronic liver disease, loss of appetite, dryness of the mouth, alcoholic cirrhosis, cervical spondylosis, bloodshot eyes, nose bleeds, hepatitis, bitter taste in the mouth, headaches caused by the constant consumption of alcohol, clears constipation.
- **The Great Precious Iron Pill** (*Rinchen Chags-Ril Chen-mo*)
  This precious pill contains 25 different precious gems, minerals, metals and herbs. It is wrapped in a navy blue silk cloth.
  Use & Action – treats conjunctivitis, cataracts, blurred and double vision, short and long sighted eye problems, strengthens the optic nerves, abnormal visual intolerance of light, involuntary blinking of the eyes.
- **Coral 25** (Rinchen Byur-Dmar Nyer iNga)
  Composition – coral, pearl, lapis, mother of pearl, vermilion, yellow ochre, fossils, calamine, brain-shaped stone, myrobalan, costus, sweetflag, aconite, musk, clove, nutmeg, magnet, eaglewood, asterdiplostephroides, quince, sesame seeds, felwort, saffron, liquorice, chrysanthemum, crystal sugar. It is wrapped in a pink silk cloth.
  Use & Action – treats neurological diseases, vertigo, meningitis, facial paralysis, cervical spondylosis, paralysis, encephalodynia, rigidity and contraction of the limbs, loss of balance.

All the above mentioned precious pills have great potential to treat many modern diseases but because of the laws in this country I am unable to prescribe a few of them.

HOW TO TAKE PRECIOUS PILLS

Around the time of dusk the night before taking the pill, unwrap it from its cloth and put it in an unbroken and clean porcelain cup (this is a symbol of good health), and pour half a cup of boiling hot water into it. The cup should be covered with a small plate, not exposed to any light, and left to soak overnight. The patient also has to separately soak seven Tibetan peppers called *yer-ma* and then boil them into a decoction which is strained and drunk that evening. This will help to open all the subtle pathways of the channels. Ten saffron stalks are also soaked separately and left overnight.

The following morning the patient gets up early and washes thoroughly. Warm water is then added to the precious pill mixture from the night before and then it is stirred with the ring finger until it has dissolved. It is also very good to recite the Medicine Buddha mantra (*Tadyatha Aum Bhaishjya Bhaishjya Maha Bhaishjya Bhaishjya Raja Sa-Mud-Ga-Te Svaha*) seven times while doing this. The mixture should be drunk without leaving any sediments or particles in the cup. The saffron liquid is then strained and drank as this helps to close the subtle pathways of the channels. After taking the precious pill the patient should go to bed for an hour wrapped up in warm clothes.

The day before taking the precious pill and the day after all forms of alcohol, garlic, onions, meat, fish and eggs should be avoided. Strenuous physical exercise and sexual intercourse must also be avoided. The best day on which to take a precious pill is a full moon day or on another auspicious day according to the Tibetan lunar calendar. If it is an emergency the precious pill can be taken immediately but the effect will not be so great.

PRECAUTIONARY ADVICE

It is possible to buy precious pills in India and Nepal. However, it is very important to buy them from a recognized source such as a branch clinic of the Tibetan Medical and Astrological Institute, or a well-known and respected private clinic. There are many fake precious pills which are packaged in exactly the same manner as the authentic ones and therefore it is best to avoid buying them from market stalls and private shops. Generally the Tibetan Medical and Astrological Institute does not sell more than two per person of the most powerful precious pills (unless more have been prescribed by a physician). This is because of the length of preparation involved in the making of genuine precious pills and their limited supply.

10) HERBAL COMPOUNDS

There are 42 herbal compounds mentioned in the medical texts. It is said that at the end of aeon when all the precious resources of the earth have been used, there will only be herbal compounds left to treat people. Wherever we go in the world there are medicinal herbs growing which can be used if we are able to recognize them. Because of this we have a special chapter on herbal compounds in the medical texts.

ARE THERE ANY SIDE EFFECTS OF TAKING TIBETAN MEDICINE ?

There are 12 adverse effects if the physician was not fully qualified, or the medicines were not manufactured following the proper procedures.

1 *Loong* treatment in excess pacifies *Loong* but aggravates *mKhris-pa*.
2 *Loong* treatment in excess pacifies *Loong* but aggravates *Bad-Kan*.

3 Due to wrong treatment *Loong* is not pacified and gives rise to *mKhris-pa*.
4 Due to wrong treatment *Loong* is not pacified and gives rise to *Bad-Kan*.
5 *MKhris-pa* treatment in excess pacifies *mKhris-pa* but aggravates *Loong*.
6 *MKhris-pa* treatment in excess pacifies *mKhris-pa* but aggravates *Bad-Kan*.
7 Due to wrong treatment *mKhris-pa* is not pacified and gives rise to *Loong*.
8 Due to wrong treatment *mKhris-pa* is not pacified and gives rise to *Bad-Kan*.
9 *Bad-Kan* treatment in excess pacifies *Bad-Kan* but aggravates *Loong*.
10 *Bad-Kan* treatment in excess pacifies *Bad-Kan* but aggravates *mKhris-pa*.
11 Due to wrong treatment *Bad-Kan* is not pacified and gives rise to *Loong*.
12 Due to wrong treatment *Bad-Kan* is not pacified and gives rise to *mKhris-pa*.

THERAPIES

There are various therapies in Tibetan medicine and described here are those which are most relevant. Performing therapy can be categorized into two: rough therapy and mild therapy. Rough therapy includes blood-letting, moxibustion, golden needle therapy and cupping. Mild therapy includes compresses, fomentation and ointment.

ROUGH THERAPIES

BLOOD-LETTING (GTAR-GA).

In Tibetan medicine there are 77 blood-letting points: 21 points for the head and neck, 34 for the arms, 18 for the legs, two for the stomach and two for the penis.

Blood-letting is suitable for *mKhris-pa* diseases and blood disorders such as leprosy, gout, ringworm, erysipelas, lymph disorders, body wounds and contagious fevers. It is not suitable for pregnancy, post-natal conditions, oedema, consumption, lack of digestive heat, people with a weak bodily constitution, children under 16, adults over 70, *Loong* and *Bad-Kan* disorders.

There are preliminary preparations to be made before blood-letting. Three or five days before it is performed the patient should take three different decocotions (made out of myrobal-an, moonseed, elecampane, and long pepper) to separate the pure and impure blood. On the day of blood-letting the patient should keep warm and stay in the sun to improve their blood circulation. The blood vessels in the part of the body where the letting is going to be performed should then be tightened for easy incision.

Impure blood is thin, yellowish, full of mucus and pus. When blood-letting is performed the blood flows very forcefully. If the blood is dark black and lines are visible, it means that the patient needs a herbal decoction to separate the pure and impure blood before further letting can occur. If the blood is black, coarse and its foam is red it means that the patient has a *Loong* disorder. If the blood is yellowish, thin and has a pus odour then it means the patient has a *mKhris-pa* disorder. If the blood is light, red, thick and smooth then it means the patient has a *Bad-Kan* disorder. If the blood is as red as a red lac it means that it is good blood and if this blood is produced during blood-letting the procedure must be stopped and not a drop should be wasted as this blood sustains our life.

If the disease is connected with the upper part of the body, blood is let from the jugular and redial veins. If the disease is connected with the middle part of the body blood is let from the mediociphalic and basilic veins. If the disease is connected with the lower part of the body blood is let from the saphenous and tibial veins.

The instrument used in blood-letting has to be a lancet shaped like a sparrow's feather, curved like a crescent moon and six finger widths in length. Or it should be a 'supine-shaped' lancet. The blade should be sharp enough to shave hair and it should be made by the most skilled blacksmith using the best refined iron available.

The benefits of blood-letting are that it eliminates impure blood, strengthens nerves, reduces pain, reduces swelling and inflammation, and dries up pus. In Tibetan medicine blood-letting is considered to be the best therapeutic technique. It is important that it is performed by an experienced physician otherwise it might have the reverse effect.

MOXIBUSTION

In Tibetan medicine there are 71 points for placing moxa – 20 on the posterior side of the body, 22 on the anterior side of the body, 29 on the head and limbs.

The best time to collect the edelweiss flowers which are used in moxibustion is in the autumn. This flower (in Tibetan called *trah-wah*) is anti-inflammatory, coagulant, an anti-toxin, stops bleeding and reduces swollen glands. The flowers should be thoroughly dried and made into the shape of a small cone so that it can easily remain at the related points. The small cone is then lit and left until it has completely burnt out, its size depends on the disease being treated. Fresh garlic must also be crushed and placed on the skin in order to hold the edelweiss and for its antisceptic qualities.

Moxibustion is very beneficial for *Loong* and *Bad-Kan* disorders, such as indigestion, lack of digestive heat, oedema, tumours, madness, dementia and nerve disorders. It can also dry up serum, improve bodily heat and enhance memory. It is not good when performed directly on the five senses or genitalia points. It is not good for *mKhris-pa* and blood disorders.

Moxibustion is performed on selected anterior and posterior points in the body. The main anterior moxibustion points, and benefits from placing moxa on them, are:

- The crown of the head and anterior fontanelle points – treats vertigo and *Loong* disorders.
- Nape – treats mental disorders.
- Sternum point – treats madness and depression.
- One inch below the xiphoid point is the tumour point – treats stomach tumours.
- One inch below the navel, to the left, centre, and right are the upper intestine points, and one inch below these to the left, centre, and right are the lower intestine points – all these points treat diarrhoea caused by the disturbance of *Loong*.
- Suprasternal point – treats hiccups, blockages of the throat, and eases dislocation of the heart.
- Big toes point – treats stiffness of the neck and swollen testicles.
- Middle of the left and right shoulder points – treats nose bleeding.

For the posterior points it must be noted that the Tibetan medical system counts the vertebrae on the spine using a different method to the Western system. The seventh vertebrae of the Western system in the Tibetan medical system is counted as the first vertebrae. The moxa points listed here follow the vertebrae according to the Tibetan system.

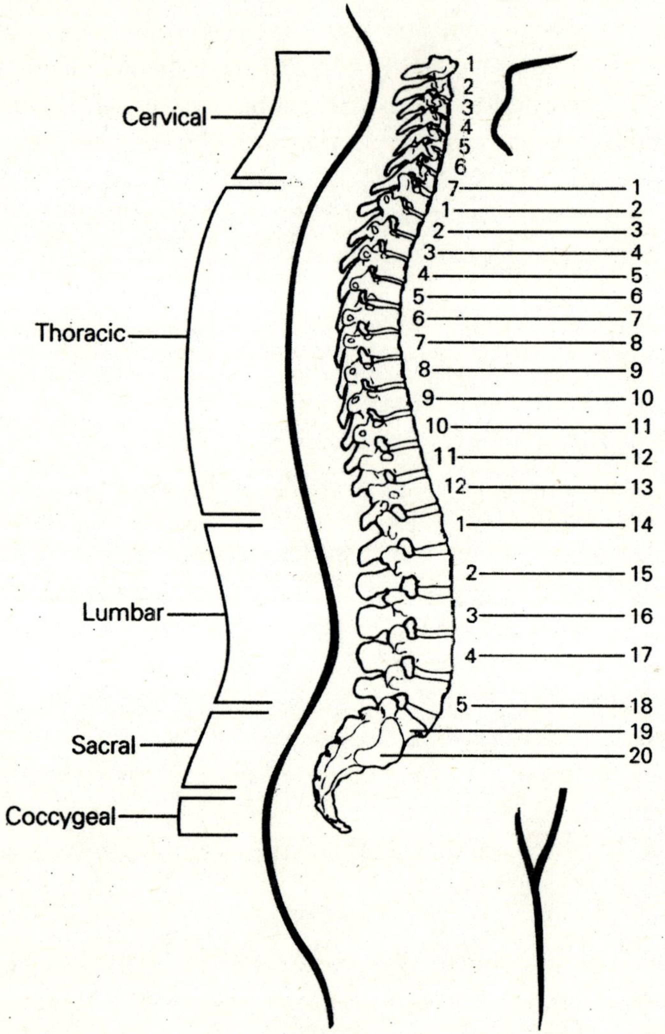

Posterior moxa points

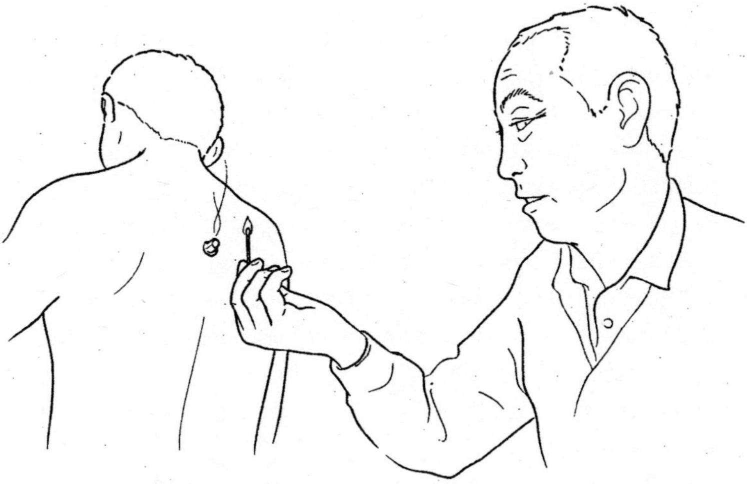

Seventh posterior moxa point for the heart

The posterior points and benefits from placing moxa on them are:

- This first vertebrae is a *Loong* point – helps mental disorders and loss of speech.
- The second vertebrae is a *mKhris-pa* point – helps cold *mkhris-pa*.
- The third vertebrae is a *Bad-Kan* point – treats pulmonary and heart diseases and headaches caused by cold *mKhris-pa*.
- The fourth and fifth vertebrae are for the lungs – helps pulmonary diseases related to *Loong* and *Bad-Kan* disorders.
- The sixth and seventh vertebrae are the life channel and heart points – helps relieve madness, insomnia, palpitations, heart diseases and forgetfulness.
- The eighth vertebrae is the diaphragm point and the ninth vertebrae is the liver point – helps eructation, vomiting,

blockage of the diaphragm, liver tumours, strengthens the liver.

- The tenth vertebrae is the gall bladder point – treats indigestion, yellow eyes jaundice, gallstones, loss of appetite, constant headaches and lack of digestive heat.
- The eleventh vertebrae is the spleen point – eliminates gas formation, heaviness of the body and heavy sleep.
- The twelfth vertebrae is the stomach point – treats lack of digestive heat, stomach tumours and chronic diarrhoea.
- The thirteenth vertebrae is the reproductive organs point – treats premature ejaculation, heavy periods, constipation and tumours of the uterus.
- The fourteenth vertebrae is the kidney point – helps all kidney diseases.
- The fifteenth vertebrae is the common point for the five vital and six hollow organs – helps all cold diseases connected with these organs.
- The sixteenth vertebrae is the large intestine point – treats tumours in the large intestine, flatulence, piles, urine retention and urine infection.
- The seventeenth vertebrae is the intestine point – helps small intestine tumours, chronic mucus and diarrhoea.
- The eighteenth vertebrae is the urinary bladder point – treats urinary stones, urine retention and frequency of urine.
- The nineteenth vertebrae is the reproductive fluids point – treats premature ejaculation and impotency.
- The twentieth vertebrae is the downward cleansing *Loong* point – treats incontinence of the bowels, constipation and mucus diarrhoea.

GOLDEN NEEDLE THERAPY

This is very similar to acupuncture, the only difference being the needle. In Tibetan medicine a 24-carat pure gold needle is used and the only point at which it is inserted is the crown of the head. It is beneficial for migraines related to *Loong* and *Bad-Kan* and for nerve disorders.

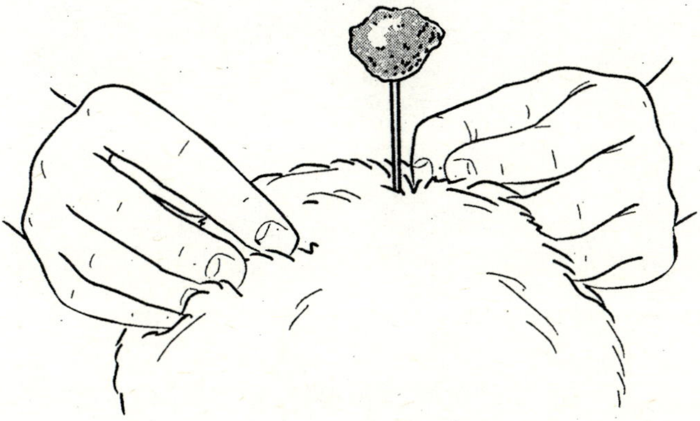

Golden needle therapy

CUPPING

Cupping is used to treat high blood pressure, relieve pain and remove damp and obstructions from the body system. The cup is made from copper as this metal helps relieve inflammation of the nerves and liver as well as heal wounds.

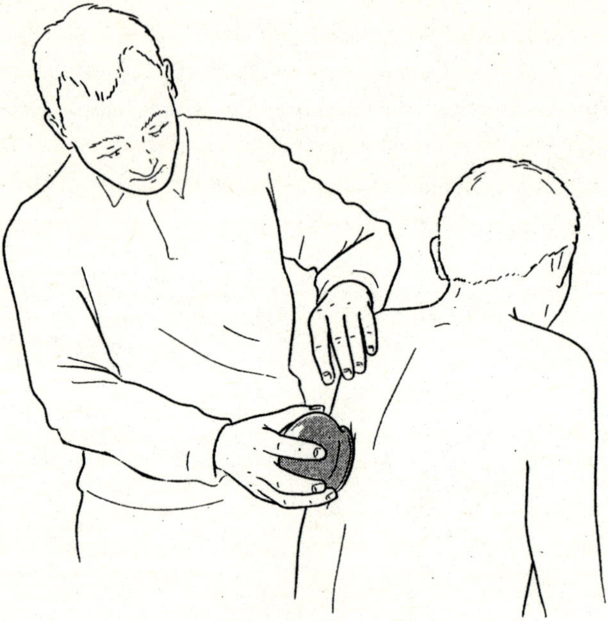

Cupping therapy

MILD THERAPIES

COMPRESSES

Compresses are divided into two: cold compresses and hot compresses. There are 11 cold and 19 hot compresses. Cold compresses include water collected beneath the stars and cold pebbles. Cold river pebbles treat imbalances of the blood and *mKhris-pa* and abdominal spasms due to fever. Black mud collected beneath the stars is used to stop nasal bleeding. Hot compresses include applying heated river pebbles and heated salt wrapped in cloth. These treat indigestion, abdominal and colon spasms.

Compresses are especially beneficial for *Bad-Kan* and *Loong* disorders, indigestion, serum disorders, abdominal and colon spasms, coagulation of the blood and pain caused by fever. They are unsuitable for oedema, advanced jaundice, leprosy or poisoning. Compresses are the most effective painkillers in Tibetan medicine.

FORMENTATION

Formentation is divided into two: bathing and wrapping formentation.

Bathing is divided into four which are connected with the five natural hot springs and wrapping is divided into 20. Wrapping formentations are a combination of medicinal ingredients such as rhododendron, juniper, ephedra, tamarisk and tansy which are mixed with water and boiled. The patient is placed in a big bath tub and allowed to soak for a long time, which helps people suffering from paralysis or from a slipped disc. It will also ease muscles, nerves, ligaments and tendons. Formentation is beneficial for lameness, muscular spasms, stiffness, gynaecological diseases, spinal deformities, serum disorders of muscle and bone tissue, chronic wounds and all problems related to *Loong* disorders. It is not suitable for oedema, people with weak bodily constitutions, loss of appetite or fully developed fever. Formentation is not advisable on the eyes, cheeks, the two big toes and the two elbows which are affected by gout, the penis, stomach and pericardium. Formentation is like a medicated sauna; the medicated steam helps to bring out all serum and impurities from the body pores. It reduces *Loong* and it reduces swelling, and after formentation a thin person puts on weight.

OINTMENTS

Ointments are divided into oil and medicinal paste applications of which there are 14 of each.

For oil application, first the oil is applied, massaged and then wiped from the skin with pea flour for the procedure to be complete. It will help to clear deposits of fats (cellulite) and clear the channels. To enhance the memory oil can be applied and massaged with melted butter; to treat eczema oil is applied with black sulphur mixed with pork fat. Sesame oil and nutmeg powder are heated up and applied on the *Loong* points such as the sternum, c-7, t-5, t-6, both the temples, both the soles and palms will help reduce *Loong* and insomnia. A combination of mustard oil and cardamom powder heated up and applied on the kidneys and back will help with regard to bedwetting.

For medicinal paste there is soot, turmeric, barberry, costus, swallow worth, buttermilk. Medicinal paste treats pimples and blemishes.

Ointments are beneficial for rough skin, deficiency of blood and reproductive fluids, weak bodily constitutions, old age, grief, mental stress, insomnia, exhaustion, retinitis pigmentosa and *Loong* disorders. They are not suitable for indigestion, gem-stone poisoning, loss of appetite, dropsy and brown *Bad-Kan* disorders.

10

CASE HISTORIES

I am sure you will be interested to read about the practical effects of Tibetan medicine. Below are a few case histories from people who I am treating and who have written to me describing the effects of the medicine.

Norma is 53 and she is a school administrator which, as you can imagine, is a very pressurized job to be in. On top of the pressures of work she is experiencing great physical change due to the menopause. She suffers from anxiety, is unable to sleep and she has weak digestion. The course of treatment which I have prescribed has been to balance her *Loong* energy and strengthen her nervous and digestive systems. She has now been taking Tibetan medicine for 13 months and here describes the effects of the medicine.[1]

> As you predicted, I found that I became calmer and less tense by following your instructions and I have now spent several weeks in a less agitated state. However, after a very relaxing half-term holiday, yesterday I suddenly became engulfed in acute anxiety, sweats and indigestion. I think this is the result of too much food from hotels and too little exercise, and I hope that when I am in my normal routine again I shall experience the more balanced state I had begun to enjoy as a result of the medicine.

Richard is 41 and a publisher. He is suffering from arthritis in his shoulders and hands. When he first came to see me his joints were so inflamed and stiff that he was unable to use his computer, which made him feel depressed. He was also taking at this time high doses of anti-inflammatory tablets. Richard has now been taking Tibetan medicine for the last 18 months and his improvement has been slow but steady; there has certainly been a significant reduction in his pain and discomfort and using a computer now presents no problem for him.

> My medicine is now almost finished and I need a refill. My arthritis is causing no real problems so that is good. I now notice that my physical and sexual energy is not as strong as usual, and if there is a way to treat this and the arthritis together that would be great!

Susan is 45 and a carer for the elderly. She is doing this work after coming out from a long meditative retreat and it has been a bit of a shock for her to lead a busy working life once again. This sudden change has caused her a lot of anxiety and she has panic attacks and palpitations as a consequence. Due to a prolonged but unbalanced vegetarian diet she suffers from lack of energy. The advice I gave her was to eat more warming and nutritious food such as fish and chicken, garlic, ginger, honey, lots of green vegetables and pulses. I advised her to avoid things which have a light and rough potency such as coffee, tea, cola, and goats' milk and cheese. She has now been taking Tibetan medicine for the last eight months and I mainly prescribed a course of treatment for her liver and for *Loong*.

> Please kindly send me two months' worth of medicine. Both the morning and evening medicines help me to relax and to boost my energy. They are both very helpful indeed so thank you very much.

Angela is 30 and she is suffering from eczema. She works in an art gallery in New York, having moved there after seeing me in London. She has been taking medicine for the last six months and I have prescribed a course of medicine to balance her *mKhris-pa* energy which is connected to the blood. I have advised her to reduce her intake of wine, citrus fruits and juices such as orange, lemon, lime and grapefruit. I have also told her to avoid anything which contains refined sugar.

> Thank you so much for sending the medicine to me. I had once again been advised by doctors here that there was nothing to be done about my terrible skin. I have sung your praises to many people here, mainly because I work with artists with HIV and AIDS and there are so many people I know that Western medicine cannot help. If you are ever visiting New York and want to hold a clinic there are many people who would book an appointment. Thank you again for all your help.

Paul is 50 and unemployed, he is suffering from arthritis, eczema and kidney disorders. Due to his weak kidneys he often has to rush to the toilet which can cause him great discomfort and inconvenience when he is out. I advised him to reduce his intake of potatoes, cold beer, sugar, citrus and cold foods; I also told him to eat more warm and cooked foods such as asparagus, cardamom, ginger, mangos and warm soups. With regard to behaviour I advised him to keep his feet and kidneys warm. He has been taking medicine for the last eight months and overall he is doing very well.

> I feel the medicine has done me wonders. I feel a lot stronger physically and mentally, also I feel much lighter and less sluggish. My skin has improved a lot and all in all there has been a great improvement. Thank you.

Shirley is 55 and an artist who suffers from bronchitis. She has constant colds and flu and has attacks of bronchitis in the cold weather. I advised her to reduce salty food such as crisps, roasted peanuts and bacon, as well as to avoid drinking chilled drinks straight from the fridge. I explained that cold and raw foods degenerate the digestive heat leading to the development of undigested particles such as phelgm and mucus which have the same characteristics of *Bad-Kan* and which cause respiratory obstruction. With regard to conduct I advised her to make sure her lungs were well protected in the cold weather as bronchitis sufferers feel much worse in cold and damp weather. She has been taking medicine for over a year and has responded very well to the treatment.

> Just a note to say thank you for giving me a year of not having bronchitis. It was wonderful not to be in bed over Christmas and New Year!

Lee is 60 and teaches English abroad. When he first came to see me he suffered from chronic liver disorder, from poor digestion and tiredness. I advised him to change his diet, particularly not to eat nuts, seeds, red meat or drink alcohol. He has now been taking Tibetan medicine for the last two-and-a-half years and overall his condition has very much improved.

> I am very happy to report that once again my liver condition is in the middle of the normal range according to my blood tests. I'm very grateful for this since, as I told you, my liver tests were abnormal for almost 23 years and they became normal for the first time when I started taking your medicine. In addition the constant slight pain in the area of my liver which used to bother me a little each day has completely disappeared.

Vinod is 47 and a civil engineer who suffers from irritable bowel syndrome, gout and kidney infections. When he first came to see me he was taking five different types of medication including sleeping pills (which he had to take due to his indigestion). I prescribed a course of medicine to treat his digestive system, gout and kidneys. With regard to diet I advised him to avoid salads and raw vegetables and citrus foods, and for him to eat his evening meal as early as possible. He has been taking medicine for six months and as soon as his stomach felt comfortable his sleep improved.

I later heard from one of his friends (who is also one of my patients) that he enjoyed dancing a *bangra* (an Indian dance) during his son's 21st birthday celebrations. This clearly showed that his gout was improving and he later told me himself that he had thrown all his previous medications in the bin.

Michael is 37 and a bank executive who suffers from pancreatitis (inflammation of the pancreas caused by viral infection) which affects his digestion of any fatty foods and when he first came to see me he was taking 13 enzyme tablets. As he leads a busy life in business it is not always easy for him to eat the correct foods. I advised him to eat fresh root ginger, coriander seeds, fennel, garlic, fish and chicken and avoid lamb, pork, alcohol and fatty foods. The medicine which I prescribed was to balance his digestive *mKhris-pa* (which is located in the small intestine) and to treat his gall bladder. He has been taking the medicine for over two years and now he only needs to take three enzyme tablets and his friends have commented on how much better he now looks.

Jean is 43 and when she first came to see me her feet were always cold and she often suffered from colds and flu. I treated her in order to improve her blood circulation and to balance her body temperature. For the last three years she has been taking just one type of Tibetan medicine each morning, called *Pomegranate Nutrient Restorer*. Since then she has not suffered from cold and flu and her immune system is so much stronger.

11

THE PRACTISING PHYSICIAN

To heal the disease of the patient the most important person is the physician. In the second tantra of the Tibetan medical texts the whole of the 31st chapter is on the practising physician. When discussing the physician, the Tibetan medical texts have six categories:

1 Qualities of the physician
2 Knowledge of the physician
3 Definition of a physician
4 Different types of physician
5 Activities of the physician
6 Final result for the physician

QUALITIES OF THE PHYSICIAN

There are six qualities a physician must possess:

1 The analytical mind which has learnt the four medical tantras and has developed some intuitive knowledge.
2 Compassion: possessing a good heart to treat all patients equally, as if treating their own mother. If you treat a patient with genuine compassion there is definite healing

power. Otherwise, even if you are the best qualified physician, if your heart is not good there will be less success. In Tibetan society it is common for a person to go to a spiritual practitioner for a divination in order to know which doctor is right for them. This means finding one which is the most suitable and with which they have a karmic connection. There are instances where one person sees two different physicians who prescribe the same medicine and yet one is more beneficial than the other.

3 Medical ethics and commitment to their practice. They must have respect for their gurus, teachers, medical instruments and fellow physicians. They should have no revulsion when seeing the pus, blood, urine, faeces and vomit of the patient. It is very important for the physician to keep the patient's confidentiality They must consider all the medicines and medical scriptures as wish-fulfilling jewels and ensure that all the medicines have been blessed according to proper Buddhist rituals.

4 Patience: the physician must be very patient in body, speech and mind. Patience through the body is making medicine, patience through speech is by making the patient happy, relaxed and comfortable, and patience through the mind is by being alert and able to accurately diagnose and treat the disease of the patient.

5 Effort and concentration: continuous effort is required to learn and gain more experience, and the concentration required when seeing a patient is the same as the concentration needed by a person who is walking on a wall with a bowl of melted butter on their head, and who is threatened with death if they spill a single drop.

6 Wisdom: the physician should be gentle, approachable, contented, have a good sense of humour and helpful towards the destitute. In Tibet the tradition was that there

was no fixed price for treatment and medicines prescribed by the physician. If the patient was rich they would offer gold, silver, horses and other fine possessions. If the patient was middle class they would offer money and if the patient was poor the treatment was free. Because of this throughout Tibetan history no poor patient has died from disease simply because they could not afford to pay for the medication.

KNOWLEDGE OF THE PHYSICIAN

The physician should know by heart the causative factors of diseases and their proper treatment.

DEFINITION OF A PHYSICIAN

The description of the physician is one who heals all pain and practises medicine to promote good health. In the reign of Songtsen Gampo (the eighth century Tibetan king) doctors were known as *Lha-je*, the king's king. In Tibetan there is a saying that although you do not wish to bow to a physician you have to, as you do not know when you might need their help. Illness afflicts rich or poor with no discrimination.

The different types of physician are divided into topmost, special and ordinary. The topmost are like the Medicine Buddha, possessing omniscient knowledge. The special possess intuitive knowledge and they are able to generate strong compassion to help the suffering of the patient. The ordinary physician must have an authentic link with their teacher, otherwise they resemble a fox seizing a king's throne – without a link with a teacher there will be no respect.

The physician must have studied the Four Medical Tantras, otherwise it is like showing material objects to someone who is blind – they will not know how to treat and diagnose disease.

A physician with no skills or experience is like someone on an unknown path – they will have no confidence and they will be full of doubt.

A physician who is unable to diagnose illness is like someone wandering in a foreign country without friends – they will be unable to distinguish a single disease.

A physician who is unable to read the pulse or perform urinalysis is like a spy unable to send their secret message – the physician will not know whether the patient has a cold disease or a hot disease.

A physician who is unable to comment on, or predict the outcome of disease is like a chieftain who cannot give a speech to his clan – the physician will gain a bad reputation.

A physician who does not know how to treat their patient resembles someone who shoots at a target in the dark – they are unable to get any response from their efforts.

A physician with no knowledge of diet and conduct is like a king who is opposed by his subjects – the patient eats the wrong food and does the wrong things which in turn weaken their bodily constitution.

A physician who cannot prepare medicine is like a farmer who does not how to cultivate the land – wrongly prepared medicine can disturb the whole system and cause various side effects.

A physician who cannot prepare cathartic medicinal compounds is like someone pouring water onto sand where nothing will come out – if emetics are being used they are not working.

A physician with no medical instruments or who is without medicine is like a courageous warrior going to war with no weapons – the physician is unable to eliminate any diseases.

Finally the physician who has no knowledge of blood-letting and moxibustion is like a thief in a house who has no knowledge of where the valuable things are stored – the physician cannot use the moxibustion and blood-letting points of the body.

The medical texts say that is important to avoid such physicians, who are said to be like demons of death in the guise of doctors. In the context of Tibetan medicine in the West I have met people who claim they have studied Tibetan medicine merely from attending a few workshops or lectures. People should therefore be cautious and not taken in by glossy advertisements which they might see in a magazine. The best recommendation is always from a patient who has taken and benefited from the treatment. It is important to always investigate thoroughly and check on the qualifications of a physician.

ACTIVITIES OF THE PHYSICIAN

Physically they should try to collect as much medicine as possible in order to prescribe the right kind of medicine for disease. They always think about the needs of the patient and they should always be available. Verbally they should be able to predict whether the disease of the patient is curable or not. Mentally they should possess the six perfections of generosity, ethics, patience, effort, concentration and wisdom.

THE RESULT OF PRACTICE

The short-term results of being a good physician are that you will be happy as it is one of the most rewarding professions in which you will meet many wonderful people from all walks of life. If you practise ethically it is said in Tibetan that a good doctor will never starve and will gain many good friends.

The long-term results of being a good physician are that if you are fully motivated and concentrated on healing patients you will achieve enlightenment in this life just through treating patients.

Commiting one's life to medicine is the most practical way of helping others. His Holiness the Dalai Lama once told his personal senior physician Dr Tenzin Choedrak that it was not necessary for him to spend his time doing religious practice. Rather it was far more important for him to spend his time researching and developing new forms of medicine to relieve the human sufferings of the modern age.

FINAL THOUGHTS

MEDICINAL BUDDHA PRAYER

I hope the reader will have gained some understanding of Tibetan medicine through reading this book. I pray that Tibetan medicine will contribute towards the relief of the suffering of all sentient beings. This is the medicinal Buddha prayer –

Homage to Buddha Vaiduryaprabha
Transcendent One compassionately acting on
Behalf of living beings,
The mere hearing of whose name offers sanctuary
From the sufferings of inferior existences,
Spiritual master of medicine, dispelling diseases
Caused by the three poisons –
Attachment, aversion and delusion.

RESOURCES

USEFUL ADDRESSES

INDIA

Tibetan Medical and Astrological Institute
Gangchen Kyishong
Dharamsala 176215
District Kangra (H.P.)
INDIA
Tel : 00 91 1892 226118
Fax : 00 91 1892 24116
Email : tmai@dsala.tibetnet

Dr Yeshi Dhonden
Ashoka Niwas
Mcleod Ganj
Dharamsala 176215
District Kangra (H.P.)
INDIA
Chagpori Tibetan Medical Insititute
Trogawa House
North Point
Darjeeling 734104

West Bengal
INDIA
Tel / Fax : 00 91 0354 70266

TIBET

Lhasa Men-Tsee-Khang
Outpatients Clinic
10 Yu Tuo Road
Lhasa
TIBET

UNITED STATES

Dr Choyang Phuntsok
Institute of East West Medicine
102 E30th Street
New York City
NY 10016
UNITED STATES
Tel : 00 1 212 683 1221
Fax : 00 1 212 683 1983

Dr Dickey P. Nyerongsha
1200 Keith Avenue
Berkeley
CA 94708
UNITED STATES
Tel : 00 1 510 843 5630
Fax : 00 1 415 647 1621

Dr Lobsang Rapgay
UCLA
2206 Benecia Avenue
Westwood

CA 90064
UNITED STATES
Tel : 00 1 310 282 9918
Fax : 00 1 310 282 3424
Email : Lobsang@ucla.edu

GERMANY

Dr Namgyal Qusar
Steyrer Str 11
Freiburg
79117 GERMANY
Tel : 00 46 761 66814

HOLLAND

NSTG / TMAI
Prinsengracht 200
Amsterdam
1016 MD
HOLLAND
Tel : 00 31 20 404 4747
Fax : 00 31 20 624 2810

ITALY

Dr Pasang Yonten & Dr Chung la Arya
New Yuthog Institute for Tibetan Medicine
Via Carnevali 111
Milano 20158
ITALY
Tel : 00 39 2 376 1863

BOOKS OF RELATED INTEREST FROM NAB

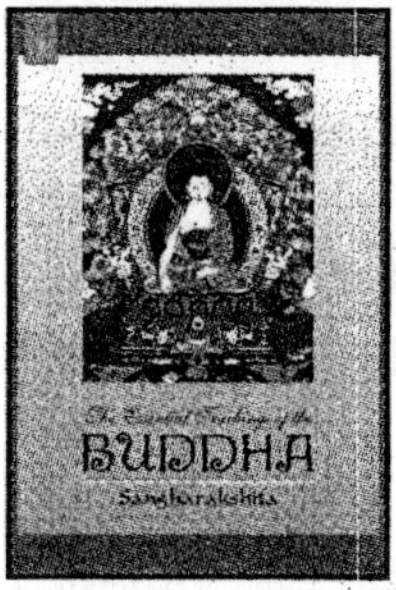

THE ESSENTIAL TEACHINGS OF THE BUDDHA—*Sangharakshita*

Refreshing, unsettling and inspiring, this book lays before us the essential Dharma, timeless and universal: The Truth that addresses the deepest questions of our hearts and minds and the Path that shows us how we can renew our lives.

ISBN: 978-81-7822-270-7

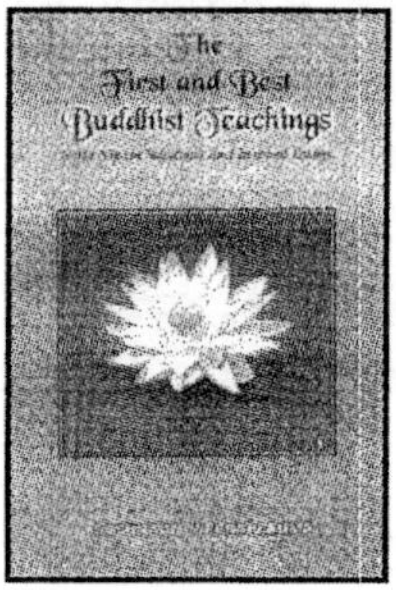

THE FIRST AND BEST BUDDHIST TEACHINGS—*Susunaga Weeraperuma*

Sutta Nipata is the oldest sacred book in Buddhist literature and is considered an authentic version of Buddha's discourses. The author's rendering of the Sutta Nipata deepens our understanding of the teachings. He lucidly expresses his understanding of this ancient wisdom in the idiom of our time. Great philosophical and psychological insights abound in this collection of essays. There are additional essays that address various issues like depression, facing death, growing old etc.

ISBN: 978-81-7822-257-8

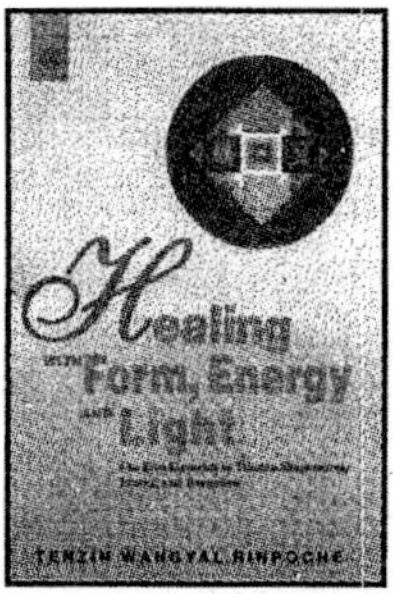

HEALING WITH FORM, ENERGY AND LIGHT—*Tenzin Wangyal Rinpoche*

Healing with Form, Energy and Light offers the reader healing meditations and yogic practices on each of these levels.Tenzin Rinpoche's purpose in this book is to strengthen our connection with the sacred aspect of the natural world and to present a guide that explains why certain practices are necessary and in what situations they are effective.

ISBN: 978-81-7822-101-4

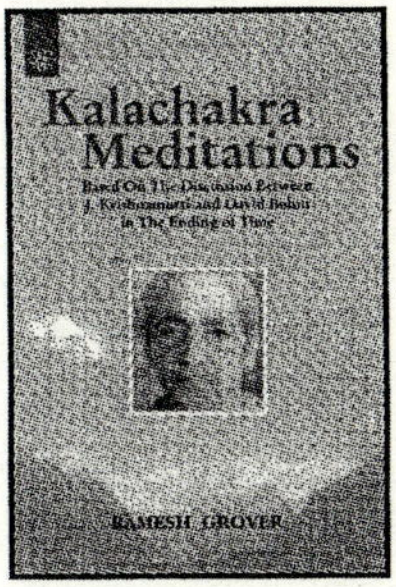

KALACHAKRA MEDITATIONS: Based on the Discussion Between J.Krishnamurti and David Bohm in The Ending of Time—*Ramesh Grover*

This book is based upon an actual meditative processing of the author's memory recall, and will be of use to others in keeping a watch, attending to what their mind perceives and reaching out to an understanding of the mischief of thought in perpetuating the delusion of 'I'. The author shares not only his joys and sorrows, as he moves within the movement of time and thought, but also, his feel of freedom in the 'ending of psychological time'. There is thus, a perception of the truth of freedom.

ISBN: 978-81-7822-279-0

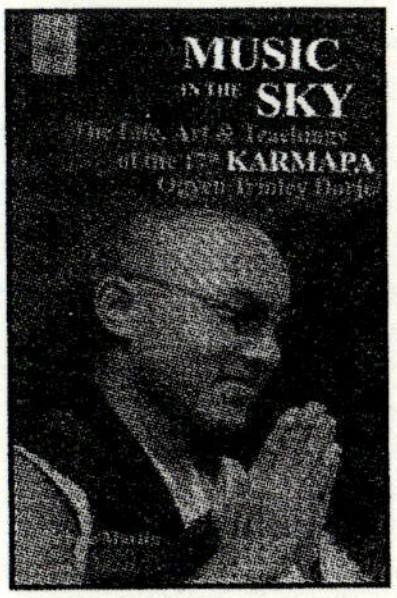

MUSIC IN THE SKY : The Life, Art & Teachings of the 17th Karmapa Ogyen Trinley Dorje
—*Michele Martin*

Music in the Sky offers a series of the Karmapa's profound teachings, an extensive selection of his poetry, and a detailed account of his life and flight from his homeland. The amazing teaching and writing skills evident in this work—particularly in light of the fact that Karmapa is still only 17 years old—will captivate readers.

ISBN: 978-81-7822-193-9

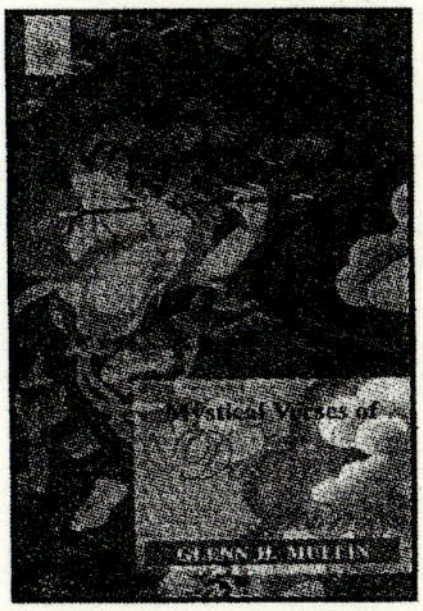

MYSTICAL VERSES OF A DALAI LAMA
—*Glenn H. Mullin*

The Tibetan tradition of mystical verse is brought stunningly to life by renowned translator Glenn Mullin through these spontaneous outpourings of the ecstasy of enlightenment. Step into the visionary life of the outspoken and unconventional Second Dalai Lama, who was "crazed" by the wisdom of the nature of reality.

ISBN: 978-81-7822-117-5

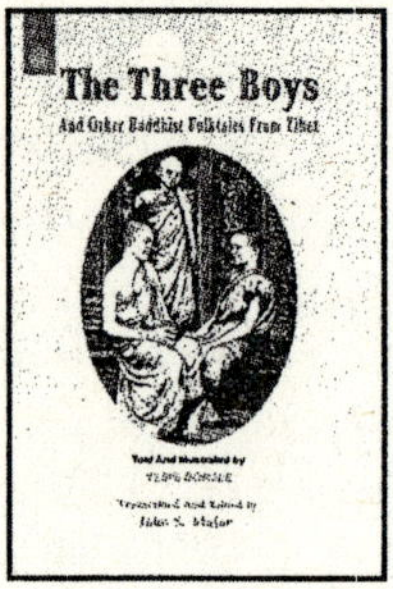

THE THREE BOYS: And Other Buddhist Folktales From Tibet—*Yeshi Dorjee & John S. Major (ed.)*

A virtuous young woman journeys to the Land of the Dead to retrieve the still-beating heart of a king; a wily corpse-monster tricks his young captor into setting him free; a king falls under a curse that turns him into a cannibal; a shepherd who understands the speech of animals saves a princess from certain death. Fifteen stories are told for modern readers in a vivid, accessible style that reflects a centuries-old tradition of story telling in the monastories and marketplaces of Tibet.

ISBN: 978-81-7822-351-3

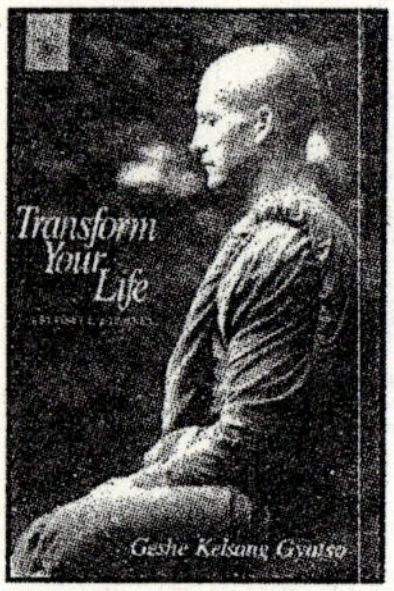

TRANSFORM YOUR LIFE: A Blissful Journey
—*Geshe Kelsang Gyatso*

By using our human life for gaining spiritual realization we can solve all our human problems and fulfill all our own and others' wishes. What could be more meaningful than this? By following the practical advice given in this book we can transform our mind and our life, fulfill our human potential, and find everlasting peace and happiness.

ISBN: 978-81-7822-070-3

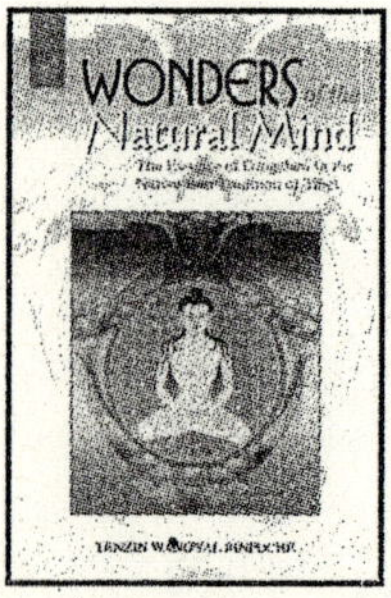

WONDERS OF THE NATURAL MIND:The Essence of Dzogchen in the Native Bon Tradition of Tibet— *Tenzin Wangyal Rinpoche*

Wonders of the Natural Mind presents the Dzogchen teachings based on the *Zhang Zhung Nyan Gyud*, the fundamental Bon text, summarizing the main points of Dzogchen and explaining its relation to the various systems of Bon teachings.

ISBN: 978-81-7822-191-5